Quality Assurance and Control in Diagnostic Radiology and Imaging

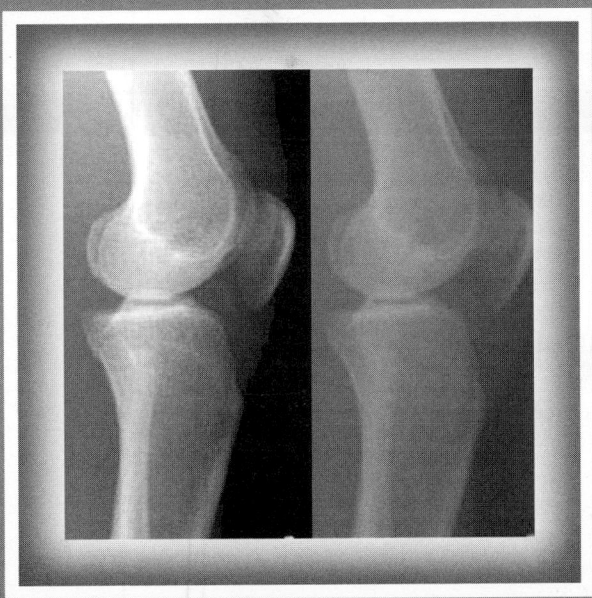

Contributors

Sumeet Bhargava DNB (Radiodiagnosis) FIAMS FCGP FIMSA FICRI
Consultant Radiologist, Kailash Hospital, Noida (UP)

Bushra Khan MSc (Medical Imaging Technology)
Tutor, Department of Radiology and Imaging, School of Medical Sciences and Research, Sharda Hospital, Sharda University, Greater Noida (UP)

Niranjan Baghel MSc (Medical Imaging Technology)
Technologist, Department of Radiodiagnosis and Imaging, Vardhman Mahavir Medical College associated Safdarjung Hospital, Delhi

Quality Assurance and Control in Diagnostic Radiology and Imaging

Satish Kumar Bhargava
MD (radiodiagnosis), MD (radiotherapy), DMRD
FICRI, FUSI, FCCP, FIAMS, FIMSA, FAMS

Professor and Head, Department of Radiology and Imaging,
School of Medical Sciences and Research, Sharda Hospital
Sharda University, Greater Noida, UP
ex-Professor and Head, Department of Radiology and Imaging
University College of Medical Sciences (Delhi University) and
associated GTB Hospital, Delhi

CBS

CBS Publishers & Distributors Pvt Ltd

New Delhi • Bengaluru • Chennai • Kochi • Kolkata • Mumbai
Hyderabad • Jharkhand • Nagpur • Patna • Pune • Uttarakhand

Quality Assurance and Control in
Diagnostic Radiology
and Imaging

ISBN: 978-81-239-2594-3

First Edition: 2015

Reprint: 2022

Published by Satish Kumar Jain and produced by Varun Jain for

CBS Publishers & Distributors Pvt Ltd

4819/XI Prahlad Street, 24 Ansari Road, Daryaganj, New Delhi 110 002, India.

Ph: 011-23289259, 23266861, 23266867 Website: www.cbspd.com

Fax: 011-23243014 e-mail: delhi@cbspd.com; cbspubs@airtelmail.in.

Corporate Office: 204 FIE, Industrial Area, Patparganj, Delhi 110 092

Ph: 011-4934 4934 Fax: 011-4934 4935 e-mail: publishing@cbspd.com; publicity@cbspd.com

Branches

- **Bengaluru:** Seema House 2975, 17th Cross, K.R. Road, Banasankari 2nd Stage, Bengaluru 560 070, Karnataka, India
  Ph: +91-80-26771678/79 Fax: +91-80-26771680 e-mail: bangalore@cbspd.com
- **Chennai:** 7, Subbaraya Street, Shenoy Nagar, Chennai 600 030, Tamil Nadu, India
  Ph: +91-44-26680620, 26681266 Fax: +91-44-42032115 e-mail: chennai@cbspd.com
- **Kochi:** 42/1325, 1326, Power House Road, Opp KSEB, Ernakulum, Kochi 682 018, Kerala, India
  Ph: +91-484-4059061-65,67 Fax: +91-484-4059065 e-mail: kochi@cbspd.com
- **Kolkata:** 6/B, Ground Floor, Rameswar Shaw Road, Kolkata-700014 (West Bengal), India
  Ph: +91-33-2289-1126, 2289-1127, 2289-1128 e-mail: kolkata@cbspd.com
- **Mumbai:** PWD Shed, Gala no 25/26, Ramchandra Bhatt Marg, Next to JJ Hospital Gate no. 2, Opp. Union Bank of India, Noorbaug Mumbai-400009, Maharashtra, India
  Ph: +91-22-66661880/89 e-mail: mumbai@cbspd.com

Representatives

- Hyderabad 0-9885175004
- Jharkhand 0-9811541605
- Nagpur 0-9421945513
- Patna 0-9334159340
- Pune 0-9623451994
- Uttarakhand 0-9716462459

Printed at Rashtriya Printers, Dilshad Garden, Delhi, India

Preface

Radiology is an indispensable speciality in the field of medical sciences and utilizes various radiological and imaging modalities like X-rays, special contrast investigation, ultrasound, CT scan, MRI scan, PET scan, digital radiography and subtraction angiography. To reach a definitive diagnosis for patient management with expanding horizon in the medical field and advancement, particularly in the last 3–4 decades, i.e. radiological revolution and the need of documentation of the patient condition, there is an increased requirement of radiological establishment both in public and private sectors. As the imaging modalities require sophisticated equipment to be operated by well-trained technologists, and for correct interpretation to achieve the correct diagnosis, optimal performance and quality control evaluation of the equipment is required periodically. The quality assurance (QA) program involves many activities, including control testing, preventive maintenance, equipment calibration, in-service education, acceptance testing of new equipment and evaluation of the new products. Hence proper understanding of QC and its proper implementation is very important for optimal performance of the equipment, resulting in accurate results and diagnosis.

The purpose of this book is to make aware various quality assurance tests involved in various radiological and imaging modalities in the radiology department in any hospital or medical institution. I am sure the book will definitely be beneficial not only to the technologists responsible for maintaining and handling the equipment but also the radiologists and residents.

Satish Kumar Bhargava

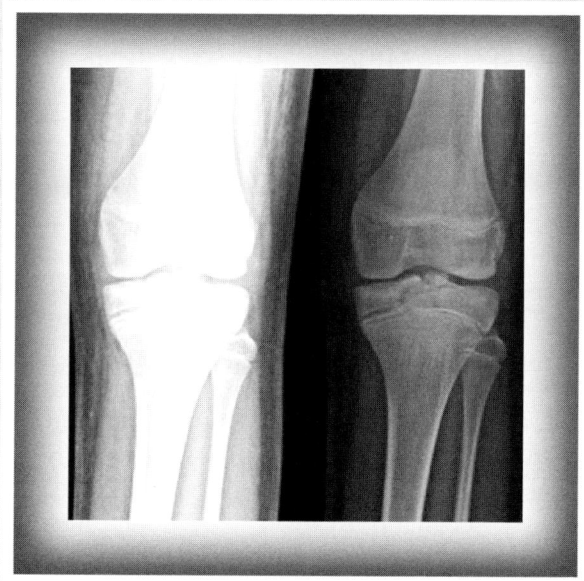

Contents

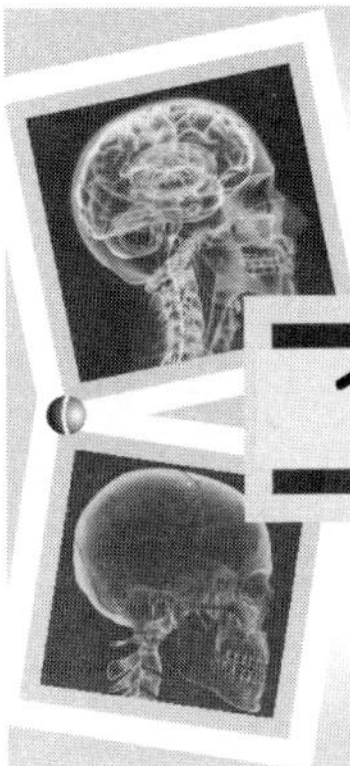

1 Diagnostic Radiology

Satish K Bhargava, Sumeet Bhargava, Bushra Khan, Niranjan Baghel

INTRODUCTION

"Diagnostic radiology facility" means any facility in which an X-ray system is used in any procedure that involves irradiation of any part of the human body for the purpose of diagnosis or visualization.

"Quality assurance" means the planned and systematic actions that provide adequate confidence, a diagnostic X-ray facility will produce consistently high quality images with minimum exposure of the patients and healing arts personnel. The determination of what constitutes high quality will be made by the facility producing the images. Quality assurance actions include both "quality control" techniques and "quality administration" procedures. "Quality assurance program" means an organized entity designed to provide "quality assurance" for a diagnostic radiology facility. The nature and extent of this program will vary with the size and type of the facility, the type of examinations conducted, and other related factors.

"Quality control techniques" are those techniques used in the monitoring (or testing) and maintenance of the components of an X-ray system. The quality control techniques thus are concerned directly with the equipment.

"Quality administration procedures" are those management actions intended to guarantee that monitoring techniques are properly performed and evaluated and that necessary corrective measures are taken in response to monitoring results. These procedures provide the organizational framework for the quality assurance program.

"X-ray system" means an assemblance of components for the controlled production of diagnostic images with X-rays. It includes minimally an X-ray high voltage generator, an X-ray control, a tube-housing assembly, a beam-limiting device, and the necessary supporting structures. Other components that function with the system, such as image receptors, image processors, view boxes, and darkrooms, are also parts of the system.

Diagnostic radiology's basic task is to provide high quality diagnostic image information about anatomic detail or ongoing physiological process within patient's body. Ensuring adequate clinical diagnostic information together with the least possible exposure of the patient to radiation (as low as reasonably achievable—ALARA principle).

Quality assurance (QA) program's main goal is optimization of radiological practice. Implementation of QA program does not mean just meeting legal requirements regarding quality control (QC) of X-ray and associated equipment and areas where they are installed but also implies the optimum use of equipment, human and material resources inspected through film rejection analysis and monitoring of patient doses received in particular radiological diagnostic examinations.

Purpose

This manual is designed to offer assistance and guidance to a radiologic technologist implementing and operating a quality assurance program in diagnostic radiology. It is designed for implementation at any level of service from a single unit that is infrequently operated to a large number of units operating at maximum capacity in a large institution.

TEST EQUIPMENT

Equipment Requirements

Many of the test tools can be made by the user. Such items include test phantoms, mesh patterns, alignment fixtures, and timing tools. Their construction is described in the text. Other test tools, such as the test cassette, require calibration and adjustment which is feasible only when a quantity can be made.

Quality Assurance Program

(a) **General considerations:** An adequate diagnostic quality assurance (QA) program involves periodic checks of the components in a diagnostic X-ray imaging system. The optimum QA program for any individual facility will depend on a number of factors which include, but may not necessarily be limited to, items such as the type of procedures performed, type of equipment utilized, and patient workload. The program should be developed under the guidance and supervision of a medical physicist qualified in this area of expertise by education, training, and experience. The qualified medical physicist should be involved in close consultation during design, initiation, implementation, and evaluation phases of the program. This program should identify the items to be monitored and establish the testing intervals. All test results should be recorded and periodic reviews of the results of the testing programs should be carried out to identify needed changes.

(b) **Room log:** An individual equipment log should be maintained on each X-ray unit in a facility. This equipment log must be kept at some convenient location where anyone using the facility (physicians, technologists, physicists, service engineer, etc.) can get ready access. The log should contain:

i. Equipment Data Specifications
   - Technical specifications, including tube loading charts.

- Equipment operating instructions.
- Detailed identification of major components of the system including name, serial number, and date of installation.

ii. An outline of the applicable quality assurance program.
iii. A log of the quality assurance test results.
iv. A record of service on the equipment including a description of system malfunctions and description of what service was carried out. The service record should also include identification of the individual performing the service and date.

(c) **Recording test data:** All quality assurance test data should be recorded on standardized forms. Examples of such forms are given in the appendix. It is suggested that each institution develops its own forms suitable to its own needs.

1. The use of standardized forms will assure that all of the required data will be obtained.
2. Forms should be filled as a part of the room log.
3. The charting of trend data is a recommended procedure which will allow easy identifications of variation with time. This is of particular value in case of film processors.

Condition of the X-ray Facility

(a) **Mechanical integrity:** A general observation of the diagnostic system should be made. Key items to look for are the presence of loose or absent screws, bolts, or other structural elements that may have been improperly installed or have worked loose due to use. The functioning of meters, dials, and other indicators should be checked. The operation of pilot lights that are often necessary to observe equipment functions in a darkened examination room should also be checked.

(b) **Mechanical stability:** To obtain a diagnostic quality radiograph, it is important to minimize patient motion.

Of key importance from the equipment side are the stability and stiffness of the X-ray tube hanger and image receptor, (i.e. table Bucky or wall mounted cassette holder). The availability and adequacy of patient support devices such as the table or immobilizing devices should also be checked. In addition it is important to check the reproducibility of positioning of the source and image receptor that may be indicated by physical marks or detents. A check of the accuracy of angulation scale should be made. As part of the check of structural stability an inspection of the electrical and/or mechanical locks on the machine should be carried out.

(c) **Electrical integrity:** The external condition of the high voltage cables should be observed. Check to make sure that the retaining rings at the termination points are tight and there are no breaks in the insulation. It is important to observe the "lay" of the cables. If they do not hang properly, they can interfere with positioning of the tube and may fail prematurely.

(d) **Electrical safety:** The system should be checked properly. This involves a physical inspection of the electrical wiring. Key areas where problems often occur include the power cord to light indicators in the beam limitation system, the wires to the exposure hand switch, and other similar power hook ups. Verify that all elements are well grounded (to each other and to the ground).

(e) **Alignment and SID:** Source to image receptor distance (SID) indicators should be checked. The consistency between multiple SID indicators (indicators on the tube support and the collimator) should be verified. The accuracy of these indicators should also be verified with a tape measure. Verification of proper grid installation should be made. This check should also include a verification of the alignment of the X-ray source and center of the grid.

(f) **The radiograph as a QA tool:** The goal of a diagnostic quality assurance program is to produce radiographs of consistent high quality, the only quality control check since acceptable radiographs can be obtained when individual elements in the system (generator, image receptor and processor) are operated outside acceptable limits. For example, compensation for inadequate film development can be corrected by unacceptable increases in exposure.

i. ***Rejected films:*** Unacceptable radiographs can result from a variety of factors that include patient motion, positioning error, improper technique selection and equipment related problems. A review of the rejected films should be made on a periodic basis to identify the magnitude of the problem and to determine the causes.

ii. ***Accepted films:*** Good practice should always question the adequacy of radiographs of less than optimal quality for their acceptability in making a diagnosis. Repeating a procedure to get a film of optimal quality is often not necessary and should be evaluated in terms of the radiation exposure and cost of retake. The need for some QA action include static marks, contrast changes and streak marks. Many other items may also be indications of less than adequate system performance. A few examples are given below:

   i. The necessity to change technique factors may indicate changes occurring in the X-ray system or development stage.
   ii. Changes in the appearance of bone or image contrast in studies where iodine based contrast media is used often indicates a shift in tube potential.
   iii. Excessive base fog in areas covered by film blockers may indicate improper film handling and/or storage.
   iv. Asymmetry of borders of collimated images

Quality Assurance Tests

The following sections describe the quality assurance tests proposed for use by radiologic technologists. Certain tests should be done daily, e.g. checks of film processing, image focus in a special procedures room. Many tests should be done on a routine or scheduled basis to be certain that changes in performance, not detected in the routine use of the apparatus, are noted so that corrective actions can be taken.

A. Film Processor Monitoring

1. ***Definition:*** Variations of chemistry (contamination, oxidation, replenishment), temperature, agitation and other factors will cause variations in the quality of processed film. Many of the variables change slowly so that daily monitoring of processor performance and plotting the results can be used to initiate corrective actions before the radiographs have decreased in diagnostic quality. Since it is normal for X-ray generators to vary in output as much as 10% from a mean value and since the high contrast of X-ray films amplifies this variation, the use of X-ray test films, i.e. wedge films, as a processor testing means is not recommended. Instead, a regulated sensitometer is used to expose a test film in the same area, the film processed at the same time each day and the operating temperatures are recorded.
2. ***Test equipment required:*** Although the parameters to be monitored may vary from facility to facility, every diagnostic radiology facility should consider monitoring the following five key components of the X-ray system:
   (a) Film-processing.
   (b) Basic performance characteristics of the X-ray unit.
   (c) Cassettes and grids.
   (d) View boxes.
   (e) Darkroom.

Examples of parameters of the above-named components and of more specialized equipment that may be monitored are as follows:

For film-processing:

- An index of speed.
- An index of contrast.
- Base plus fog.
- Solution temperatures.
- Film artifact identification.

For radiographic X-ray units, the following parameters are important:

- Reproducibility of X-ray output.
- Linearity and reproducibility of mA stations.
- Reproducibility and accuracy of timer stations.
- Reproducibility and accuracy of kVp stations.
- Accuracy of source-to-film distance indicators.
- Light/X-ray field congruence.
- Half-value layer.
- Focal spot size consistency.
- Representative entrance skin exposures.

X-RAY TUBES AND COLLIMATORS

Test all parameters at least annually.

Overload Protective Circuit Test

1. *Definition:* Many X-ray generators have circuits which prevent the operator from exceeding the ratings of the tube. System power capability is determined by setting to the maximum mA for a 0.1 second exposure at 80 kVp. This power may be limited by the tube rating. System power is important since it determines the minimum exposure time for a given mAs. It thus has a direct relation to patient motion. A check of system power also insures proper functioning of the tube protector and assures that the tube will not be damaged by accidental overloading. The set-up of the tube protective circuit involves a trade between tube life and exposure time. A

setting well below the tube power rating will increase exposure time. A longer exposure time results in increased motion unsharpness. This test does not work for falling load generators.

2. ***Test equipment required:*** Tube rating chart.
3. ***Test procedures***:
   a. Select a tube-focal spot combination (separate test for each).
   b. Set the timer for 50 ms (1/20 sec.).
   c. In 20 kVp increments, from the minimum kVp to the maximum kVp of the generator, determine the maximum tube current at which an exposure is possible. This is done by increasing the current settings until the "overload" of "exposure lockout" indicator appears. The current setting immediately below the "lockout" condition is the "maximum permitted tube current". Record the value of current.
   d. Reset the timer to 100 ms (1/10 sec.) and repeat step b.
   e. Reset the timer to 1 sec and repeat step c.
   f. Reset the timer to the maximum available time and repeat step c.
   g. Select a different tube-focal spot combination and repeat steps b–f.
   h. If applicable, select "high speed" rotation and repeat steps a–g.
   i. If serial or cine radiography is present, select an appropriate program and repeat steps a–h.
4. ***Evaluation of results:*** From the tube ratings, determine the maximum allowable tube current for each tube, focal spot, kVp and time combination selected above. The "maximum permitted tube current" should not exceed the maximum allowable tube current (obtained from the ratings). Due to the nature of equipment design, the "maximum permitted tube current" may be up to 30% less than the single exposure ratings for single exposure

settings, and up to 50% less than the single exposure ratings for serial settings. The "maximum permitted tube current" may be up to 20% less than the serial exposure ratings for serial settings. The actual acceptance current limits must be modified in many cases because most generators have discrete mA settings (e.g. 50, 100, 200, 300, ... mA) and continuous adjustments of kVp.

X-ray Generators

The accuracy of the technique indicators is crucial to the consistent production of high-quality radiographs from room to room and from patient to patient. Depending on intended use, the range of techniques to be measured may vary. For example, a generator placed in a room intended for dedicated chest radiography need only function with high accuracy between 100 and 140 kVp. The same generator used in a general radiography room must maintain its accuracy over a much wider range (e.g. 50 to 120 kVp, and at 20 to 100% rated power). Performance should be spot-checked across the entire selectable range with particular attention paid to the most commonly used techniques. All generator parameters should be evaluated at acceptance and at least annually thereafter.

Exposure Time

The generator should be capable of terminating the exposure after a preselected time interval. Single-phase units may only be capable of terminating an exposure in increments of 8.3 ms (assuming a 60 Hz power source). Three phase and mid-frequency generators should be capable of accurately terminating the exposure after 2 ms and at virtually any time interval thereafter (forced extinction). For generators that display the selected time prior to the exposure, accuracy should be within ±5% (for times greater than 10 ms) and ±10% for time less than 10 ms. Reproducibility of the exposure time should be within a coefficient of variation <0.05.

Definition: This test procedure describes the use of a spinning top to determine the accuracy and reproducibility of the timer settings on single phase, three phase, and constant potential radiographic X-ray units. For the purpose of this test procedure, accuracy will mean the degree of agreement between the measured and indicated time values. Reproducibility will mean the degree of agreement between several measurements of the exposure time at the same indicated time on the X-ray control panel. The accuracy and reproducibility of the timer stations on diagnostic X-ray equipment are important because they directly affect the mAs and hence the amount of radiation emitted. Poor timer reproducibility will result in erratic radiographic results which may be attributed to other causes. There are three basic types of tops used for determining X-ray exposure time: Manually energized tops, manually energized synchronous tops, and synchronous motor-driven tops. The manually energized top, the classical spinning top, is a metal (usually brass) disk with a hole or slit. If it is spinning while radiographed using a single phase X-ray generator, the resulting radiograph will show a distinct black dot for each 1/120 sec pulse of the X-ray unit. Counting the number of pulses delivered in the test exposure yields the measured exposure time.

For basic performance characteristics of the X-ray unit

X-ray Output and Beam Quality

The beam quality has a major impact on patient dose and a smaller impact on the quality of the final image. Beam quality will change as the X-ray tube ages due to deposition of target material on the inside of the tube window and to roughening of the target track. This measurement should be made at least annually and whenever the X-ray tube or collimator is replaced or serviced.

1. ***Definition:*** The output and beam quality are evaluated using a fixed and reproducible geometry. The output of a system may change as a result of component failure,

absence of a required filter, drift from calibrated values or other causes. The beam quality test verifies that the half-value layer is sufficient to reduce patient exposure to low-energy radiation and assures that filters, which may have been removed for mammography or tube inspection, are in place for normal radiography.

2. ***Equipment required:***
   (a) Radiation detector (low energy), either a direct-reading pocket dosimeter or an ionization chamber with no active area dimension greater than 3 inches and having a suitable means for reading exposure.
   (b) Distance-measuring device such as common tape measure.
   (c) Aluminium (1100 alloy) sheets; 1 mm. 5 @ 4 in × 4 in × .04 (10 cm × 10 cm × ...)
3. ***Test procedure:***
   (a) Center the X-ray source assembly over the table.
   (b) Position the tube 100 cm above the tabletop using the system scales. Verify using the tape measure.
   (c) Adjust the X-ray field to approximately 6 in × 6 in (15 cm × 15 cm) tabletop.
   (d) The radiation detector is zeroed and placed in the center of the X-ray field on the tabletop.
   (e) At 80 kVp, adjust the mA to give approximately 2/3rd full scale reading on the radiation detector. This may require experimentation to get the required exposure reading. Record the technique factors (mA and time).
   (f) The exposure in mR is read from the detector and recorded. Repeat for a total of three exposures and record the average.
   (g) Two pieces of aluminium 1.0 mm thick are taped to the face of the collimator to intercept all of the X-ray field.
   (h) The radiation detector is zeroed and placed in the center of the X-ray field on the tabletop.

(i) The radiation detector is exposed (one exposure). The exposure with filter is recorded. Repeat for a total of three exposures and record the average.

(j) Repeat for 3.0, 4.0, and 5.0 mm total respectively.

Evaluation of Results

(a) Output for single phase machines should be about 4.0 ±1.5 mR/mA (divide dosimeter mR by exposure mA) and about 6.0 ±2 mR/mA for 3 phase machines. High or low values may indicate too little or too much aluminium filtration, a defective tube anode or miscalibration.

(b) Plot the results of steps (f) and (j) as output in mR/mA vs thickness of aluminium added. It is required for all systems that 2.3 mm Al reduces the beam by less than 50% at 80 kVp, i.e. the HVL is greater than 2.3 mm Al. In practice, most single phase machines will exceed 2.7 mm Al HVL and three phase machines will exceed 2.9 mm.

Beam Quantity (mR/mA)

The radiation output in milli-roentgens (mR) per milli-ampere second (mAs) can aid in the preparation of manual

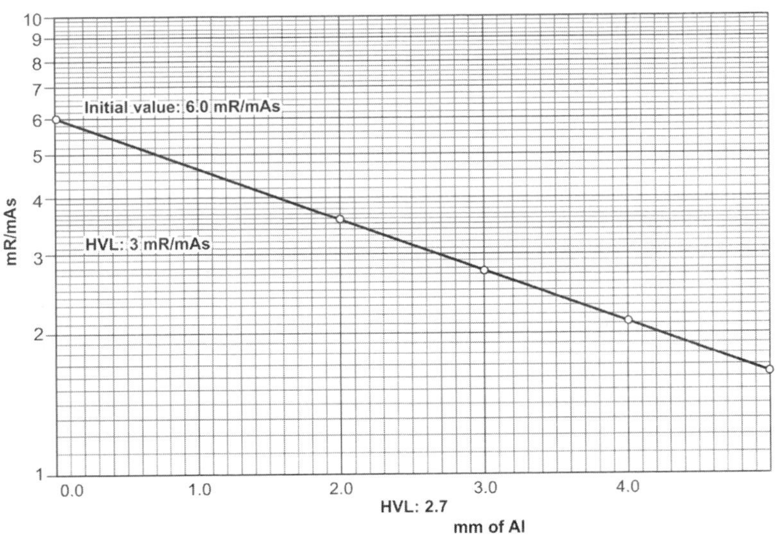

technique charts and in the calculation of patient exposure. Consistency of Beam Quantity with varying mA is indicative of the tube current calibration when minor fluctuations in kV are simultaneously monitored and appropriate corrections made. For constant load generators, the operating mA will depend upon the selected kV and the power rating of the tube or generator and may not be indicated on the control console. Beam quantity at adjacent mA stations is required to be within ±20% under federal law. The output should also be reproducible to within a coefficient of variation of <0.10.11. Since this quantity is indicative of proper tube current calibration, it is the task group's recommendation that the mR/mAs for all tube current settings on any given focal spot at any voltage setting be constant across the entire range of tube current settings available for that focal spot to within ±20%. Fluctuations in kV should be monitored and corrected for. Radiation output should be characterized at a variety of kV and mA settings that encompass the useful range of the system on both focal spots.

Automatic exposure control (AEC)—the AEC system should ideally provide constant optical density regardless of kV selected, mA selected, or patient thickness being imaged. An AEC device automatically terminates the exposure based upon the transmitted radiation detected by a radiation monitor placed either behind the grid or behind the image receptor.

The detector signal is used to charge a capacitor until a calibrated reference voltage is achieved at which time an exposure termination signal is generated. Depending upon the characteristics of the detector and the quality and sophistication of the AEC circuitry, the system capabilities will vary considerably. The AEC system should be capable of correcting for detector and image receptor kV dependence, beam hardening, and reciprocity law failure at long exposure times.

Light/X-ray Field Congruence of Collimators

The alignment between the light and radiation field permits the technologist to position the field to expose only the anatomy of interest. Misalignment may result in unnecessary or repeat exposure. Testing should be performed at least annually on new equipment. Test frequency may need to be increased as the system ages. The functionality of the field light should be confirmed as well as the adequacy of the field illumination. The individual X-ray field and light field borders agree to within ±2% of the SID.

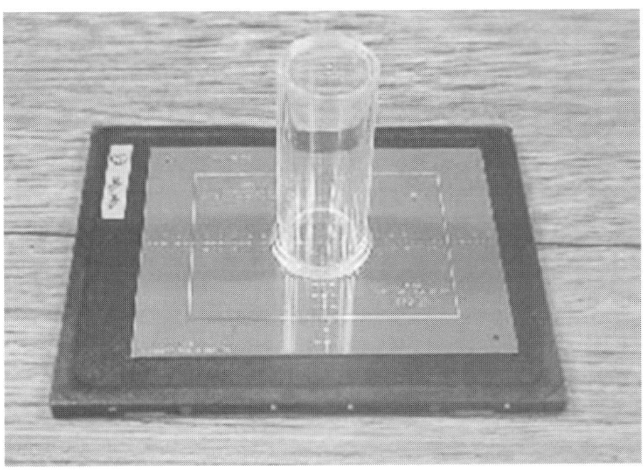

1. ***Definition:*** The purpose of the collimator light field is to allow simulation and visualization of the size, shape, and location of the field. It is important that the light field be approximately congruent to the X-ray field. Light/X-ray field misalignment may be caused by shifts in the relative positions of the light bulb filament and anode focal spot. Such shifts are caused by differences between light bulbs, shifts of mirror position, or shifts of collimator position on the tube head. This test radiographs metal strips or pennies having a known position in the light field.

2. ***Test equipment required:***

   (a) 4 each—$\frac{1}{16}$ in × 1 in × 3 in (1.5 mm × 2.5 cm × 7.5 cm) steel strips or 9 pennies or commercial alignment test tool.
   (b) 1 loaded 14 in × 17 in (35 m × 43 m) film cassette for the initial test and 8 in × 10 in (20 cm × 25 cm) for subsequent routine tests.
   (c) Common tape measure.

3. ***Test procedure:*** Initial test
   (a) Position the X-ray source over the tabletop so that the indicated distance from the source to the tabletop is 40" (100 cm) and locked in position. Verify using the tape measure.
   (b) Adjust the X-ray field size 12 in × 15 in (30 cm × 38 cm) field at the tabletop. If the system is automatically collimated, switch to manual mode. Check visually to verify that the collimator face (glass or plastic) is clean and transparent. Some collimators use a plastic filter equivalent to 1.0 to 2.0 mm Al as the faceplate. These filters often turn brown and must be replaced. Other units use thin sheet plastic as dust or safety covers and these must be intact or else replaced.
   (c) Turn on the collimator light. If necessary, dim the room light so that the edges of the light field are easily seen.
   (d) Place the loaded 14 in × 17 in cassette on the tabletop and center it in the light field.
   (e) On the top of the cassette, in the middle of each side of the light field, position one of the four metal strips so that the outer edge of the 3 inside of the strip is parallel to inside and at the edge of the light field.
   (f) A penny is used at the right shoulder position of the cassette to give the orientation of the field on the film.
   (g) Make the exposure to give a medium density ($D = 1.0$, about 60 kVp, 5 mAs).

(h) The film is then developed.
(i) The image is evaluated for misalignment of the X-ray and light fields.

4. *Test procedure:* Routine test
   (a) Position the X-ray source over the tabletop so that the indicated distance from the source to the tabletop is 40" (100 cm) and locked in position.
   (b) Place the loaded 8 in × 10 in cassette on the tabletop. Position the 9 pennies, center the cassette, and adjust the collimator so that the light field is as shown below.
   (c) Make the exposure to give a medium density (about 1.0, typ. ex.–60 kVp, 5 mAs).
   (d) Develop and inspect the film. Save the film for comparison in future tests.

Evaluation of Results

For the initial test, the misalignment (the horizontal misalignment is defined as the sum of the deviation of right and left edges, vertical as the sum of the deviation of the top and bottom edges) must each be less than line (2.5 cm). For the routine tests, the deviations should be less than ±1/2 the diameter of the penny at any edge and must be less

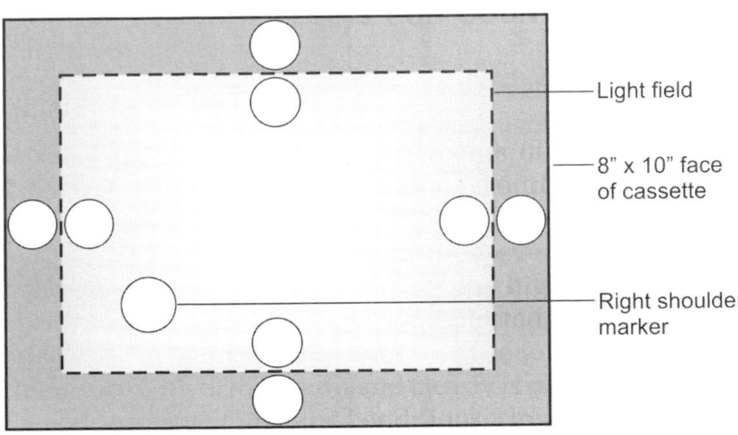

than ±1 the diameter of the penny. Commercial alignment fixtures are made with markers indicating pass-fail beam limits.

Focal Spot Size

The size of the radiation source has considerable impact upon the resolution in the image. Focal spot sizes should be measured according to National Electrical Manufacturers Association (NEMA). For general purpose imaging head and neck, abdomen, spine, long bone, genitourinary (GU) tract, etc. a good rule of thumb suggests a nominal focal spot dimension of approximately 0.1% of the SID. For detail imaging (pediatric, extremities, long bones, etc.), the measured focal spot dimensions should be less than 0.05% of the SID. These suggested specifications result in 2.0, 1.2, and 0.6 mm nominal focal spot sizes for chest, general purpose, and detail radiography, respectively. Blooming characteristics and resolving capability should be evaluated at acceptance using a star pattern.

1. ***Definition:*** The ratings of an X-ray tube are limited by the thermal properties of the anode and the geometry of the cathode structure. Generator controls usually limit the single exposure power level while other protective circuits may limit the power to the tube during multiple exposures of angiography or cineradiography. However, taking two pictures in rapid succession (single exposure ratings) or a jammed film changer may cause the system to operate beyond ratings. Operation at low kVp and high mA or holding the tube in a boosted mode too long may strain the filament. On occasion, tubes may not be identified properly. This test is not the same as the pinhole test. This test uses a metal pattern of eleven or more pairs of three bar patterns. The bars are slots in a metal mask and vary in spacing from 0.6 to 3.35 line pairs/mm or more. The bar pattern is used as a radiographic test object and images may be readily correlated to radiographic capability.

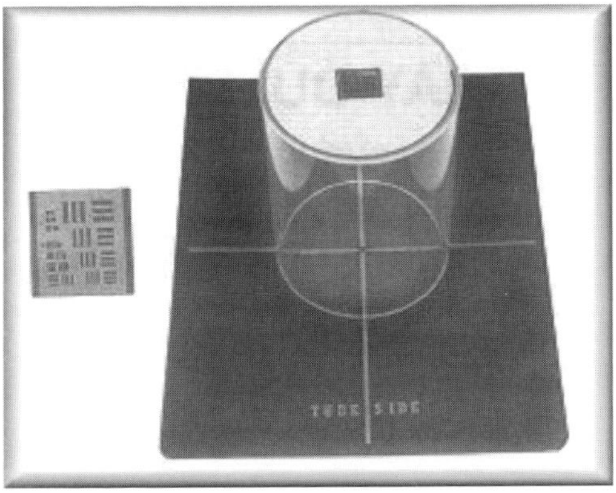

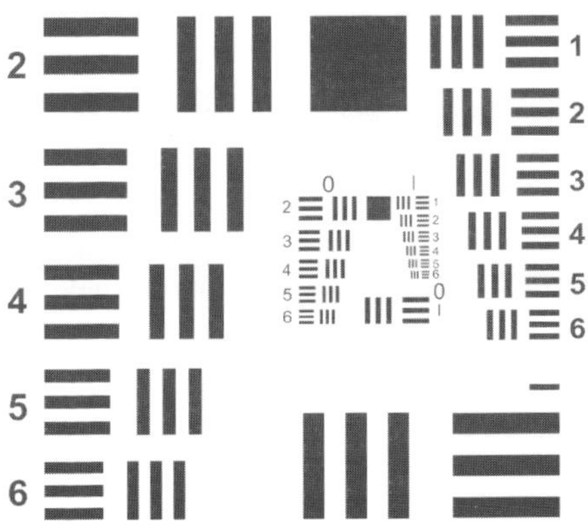

2. ***Test equipment required***
   (a) Focal Spot Test Tool consisting of a suitable bar pattern mounted in a 6 in (15 cm) test stand.
   (b) Dental Film (Kodak DF 42) or radiographic film in a cardboard cassette, non-screened.
   (c) 18 in (45 cm) scale
   (d) Aluminium plate 7 in × 7 in × 0.75 in (18 cm × 18 cm × 1.9 cm) 1100 alloy.
3. ***Test procedure:*** Center the focal spot of the tube 18 in (45 cm) above the bar pattern using the distance tape or measure 18 in (45 cm) from a point 1½ in (3.8 cm)

from the center of the tube head cylinder (estimated position of the focal spot). Place the tool over the non-screened film. Use the collimator light beam to center and confine the field to the top of the tool. Set the factors to 80 kVp and 5 to 10 mAs and expose for both focal spots, moving the film between exposures. For fluoroscopic systems, the test tool (face down) may be viewed on fluoro and shutters adjusted to display only the pattern. Place the aluminium plate on the top of the base of the test tool and fluoro at 80 kVp at 1 mA. Then place the non-screened film between the aluminium plate and the base of the test tool. Expose for 5 to 10 sec (small focus). Use an empty spot film cassette, set to 80 kVp, 5 to 10 mAs, move the film and expose (large focus). Develop the test film.

4. ***Evaluation of results:*** A group of three bars is said to be resolved when exactly three bars can be seen clearly on the film. Both of the right angle groups must be seen clearly to be resolved. The following table lists the number of groups which must be resolved. Smaller focal spot should resolve more groups.

Group Focal Spot (Nominal)

Size mm		
1.	(0.6 lp/mm)	2.0 (or smaller)
2.	(0.7 lp/mm)	2.0 (or smaller)
3.	(0.85 lp/mm)	2.0 (or smaller)
4.	(1.0 lp/mm)	2.0 (or smaller)
5.	(1.15 lp/mm)	1.8 (or smaller)
6.	(1.4 lp/mm)	1.5 (or smaller)
7.	(1.7 lp/mm)	1.3 (or smaller)
8.	(2.0 lp/mm)	1.0 (or smaller)
9.	(2.5 lp/mm)	0.8 (or smaller)
10.	(2.8 lp/mm)	0.6 (or smaller)
11.	(3.35 lp/mm)	0.5 (or smaller)

Tubes which fail to resolve the minimum number of groups should be retested with the standard pinhole test method. (Some tools will measure to 0.3 mm, refer to the supplier's instructions.)

Cassettes: Screen Speed and Film–Screen Contact

Test Frequency: **Initially and annually thereafter or as needed**

Definition: Cassettes may vary because of screens of different manufacture, age, or front panel materials. Warped cassettes, fatigue of the foam or felt compression material, worn closures, dirt, light leaks, etc., frequently produce unsharp or fogged radiographs to the point where the cassettes of screens should be replaced. Similar problems of poor film/screen contact, dirt, etc. may be present in the film changers or "cassette less" radiographic systems.

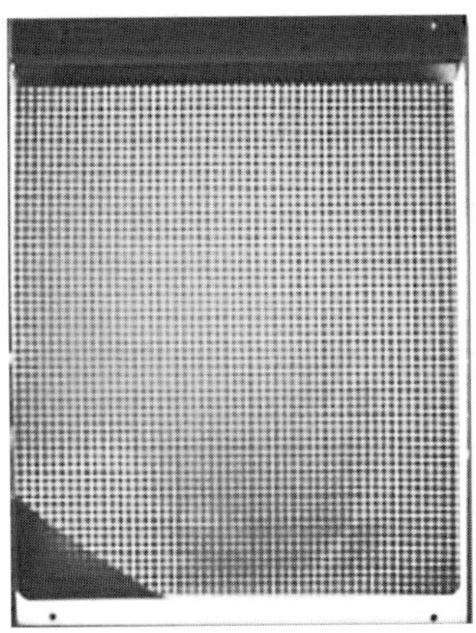

Test equipment required

(a) A 14 in × 17 in (35 cm × 43 cm) piece of 0.25 in (6 mm) galvanized wire mesh, edges taped. A 14 in × 14 in (35 cm × 35 cm) or other size pieces may be used, to check film changers. This material is available at most hardware stores as wire cloth and need not be perfectly flat.

(b) A 14 in × 17 in (35 cm × 43 cm) piece of brass wire mesh, eight mesh per inch, 0.028 in (0.7 mm) wire with 0.5 in (1.25 cm) central hole, edges taped (alternate test mesh to meet ANSI proposed standard PH1-49).

(c) A commercial tool of the appropriate size, typically 45 × 45 cm, containing a perforated metal plate to serve the same purposes as the screen or mesh tools.

Test Procedure

Physical inspection: It is not unusual after extended use to find labels missing and cassettes and screens of various speeds, age and manufacture in use without compensation, since speed differences may be unknown. Inventory and sort by intensifying screen type, age and cassette type. Relabel the cassettes to provide clear indication of the type of intensifying screen contained and redistribute the cassettes such that common types are maintained for general and/or special purposes throughout the department. Clean and inspect the intensifying screens. Look for worn areas, stained areas or yellowing due to age. Dirt specks and worn or stained areas produce artifacts on the radiographs.

Use only cleaning materials recommended by the screen manufacturer. The frequency of cleaning varies with local conditions. It is helpful to number the intensifying screens with permanent ink in an unobtrusive location and likewise to number the outside of the cassette such that a repeating artifact can be traced to a specific cassette.

Cassette–Screen Speed

If there is any doubt or question as to the equality of radiographic speeds among cassettes or screens, the following simple test should be performed. Place no more than four cassettes, preferably all the same size, on the X-ray table with corners touching; one of the four should be a known standard cassette/screen combination. All cassettes should be loaded with film from the same box. The X-ray tube is centered perpendicular to the intersection of the four cassettes, and an exposure made which will produce a film density between 0.80 and 1.50.

Screen–film contact: Lack of intimate screen–film contact within a cassette will cause lack of detail or "blurring". Film–screen contact should be tested initially before acceptance of new cassettes and screens and periodically to determine that film–screen contact is maintained in use.

A test exposure of the wire mesh is made with factors of the order of 3–5 mAs, 50 kVP, 40 inch FFD for medium speed.

Procedure: Screen–Film Contact

The procedure ensures that optimum contact is maintained between the screen(s) and film in each cassette.

Equipment Required: All Cassettes

1/8 inch mesh brass or copper screen. The mesh can be placed between two thin sheets of acrylic or cardboard to protect it.

1. Load cassette to be tested and let rest for approximately 15 minutes to allow trapped air to escape.
2. Place cassette on the table and collimate the X-ray beam to the size of the cassette.
3. Place the wire mesh screen on the top of the cassette and make an exposure. The optical density of the film should be between 1.0 and 2.0. Suggested technique is 1 or 2 mAs at 50 kVp.
4. Process the film.
5. View the film on a view box in a room with low ambient light. Stand 6–8 feet from the view box to evaluate the film.
6. Areas of poor contact will appear as dark areas or unfocused areas on the film.
7. **Record on quality control log: Annual tests maintain record for 1 year.**

Corrective Action

Areas greater than 2 cm in diameter of poor contact indicate the need for corrective action. Clean the cassettes and retest. Areas of poor contact around the periphery of the cassette may indicate faulty latches or worn seals on the cassette. If cleaning does not eliminate the areas of poor contact, the cassette should be replaced. Most cassettes have a life expectancy of 10 years with adequate care. All corrective actions must be completed within 30 days, documented and records retained for a minimum of 2 years.

Cassette Integrity

Equipment Required: All Cassettes

Cassettes must be in good physical condition in order to prevent light leaks that will fog film.

1. Examine each cassette: Cassette should be in good physical condition with no cracks, dents or other damage.
2. Check hinges: Cassette should be closed fully and easily. There should be no gaps around the edges of cassette.
3. Check latches: They should work easily to open cassette. They should close and lock easily.
4. Open cassette: Check condition of screens and grids. Screens and grids should not be cracked, broken or discolored.
5. **Record on quality control log: Annual tests and maintain record for 1 year.**

Note: If screens are damaged but cassettes are in good condition, contact service company and inquire if screen can be replaced.

Corrective Action

Replace or repair damaged cassettes immediately. If screens or grids appear damaged, they should be replaced. All corrective actions must be completed within 30 days, documented and records retained for a minimum of 2 years.

Screen Cleanliness

Equipment Required: All Cassettes

- Screen cleaner (as recommended by the manufacturer of the screens), lint-free gauze pad, equivalent lint-free cloth, or camel hairbrush.
- Canned air
   1. Visually inspect the condition of the intensifying screen.
   2. Dust the screen with the camel hairbrush and canned air.
   3. If foreign materials (e.g. dirt, developer solution) cannot be readily removed with a camel hairbrush or canned air, use liquid screen cleaner.
   4. After cleaning with manufacturer approved cleaners, screens should be allowed to air-dry, standing vertically, before returning the cassette to use.
   5. **Record on quality control log: Annual tests and maintain record for 1 year.**

Corrective Action

If the screen shows signs of cracking, fading or discoloration, it should be replaced. **All corrective actions must be completed within 30 days, documented and records retained for a minimum of 2 years.**

Screens and Film

Some experimentation may be needed to determine best exposure factors. Wire mesh radiographs should be exposed for a background density of about 1.0.

Evaluation of Results

(a) For the speed test, compare the resulting densities on the four processed test films close to the central ray. Visual densities should be the same. If a densitometer is used to compare densities, the maximum density variation should be ± 0.20.

(b) View all mesh test films from a distance of 6–8 feet (2 m); areas of poor screen/film contact will appear as dark areas or dark spots. Close inspection of these dark areas will show the wire image blurred. Small areas or poor contact around edges or in corners of the radiograph may have to be ignored.

Cassettes showing poor contact involving large areas either peripherally or centrally often offer poor prospects for repair; consider replacement. Light leaks will be evidenced by fogged edges or corners of the radiograph. This fog can generally be seen both on the screen contact radiograph and on patient radiographs. The cause may be due to faulty latches on the cassette, which may be adjusted or repaired, or due to worn light seals on the cassette or a felt light-seal that is too tight, holding the cover open, particularly on older model cassettes. Discuss indicated repair with vendor. If light leakage is severe, replacement of the cassette is indicated.

Radiographic Illuminators

1. ***Definition:*** The conditions under which a radiologist, clinician, etc. views radiographs may influence diagnostic accuracy and stamina. Viewing conditions include the brightness of the illuminators as well as the ambient room light level. Undesirable radiographic viewing conditions include:
   - (a) Low intensity illuminators.
   - (b) High ambient room-light levels.
   - (c) Gross mismatch between viewing conditions used by the radiologist and viewing conditions used by technologists to check films.
   - (d) Illuminators in the same viewing area having grossly mismatched intensities and/or color. No uniformity of radiographic illuminator brightness most commonly occurs when bulbs are replaced without regard for matching their color or intensity, and when output of the lamps change with age.

Lead aprons, gloves, gonadal and thyroid shielding integrity check

Test Frequency: Initially and annually thereafter

Standard: No breaks in protective garments

Examine the integrity of the personnel shielding devices to ensure optimal protection to the patient when positioned properly. This is a good opportunity to remind staff of the necessity of using personnel shielding on themselves and patients.

Note: Lead aprons should never be folded. Cracks in the lead lining can develop at the fold, reducing the useful life of the apron.

Do not assume that brand new aprons, gloves, etc. contain no defects. Visual examination is not sufficient to ensure integrity of shielding. New aprons, gloves, etc. should be examined under X-ray immediately upon arrival and returned to supplier if defects are found.

Equipment required: Personnel shielding devices

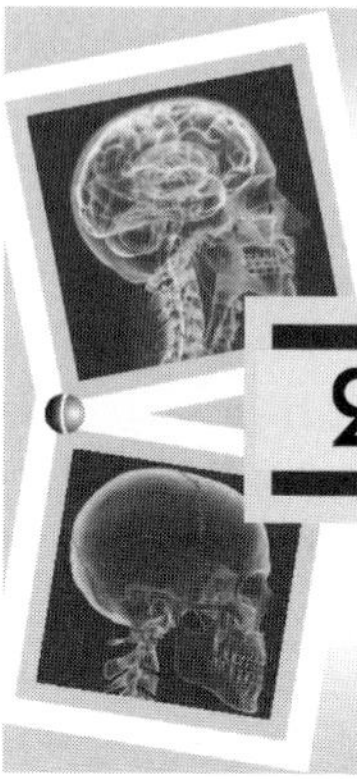

2 Quality Control in Fluoroscopic Unit

Satish K Bhargava, Bushra Khan, Sumeet Bhargava

Fluoroscopy is generally performed to aid in the positioning of medical devices within a patient, to localize sites for surgical excision, or to position the patient for static radiographs. It uses relatively low radiation dose rates, typically 10 to 80 µGy/min at the detector face. This results in rather noisy images. Fluoroscopic images are not usually recorded.

Fluorography is the acquisition of a series of high definition dynamic images. It is used primarily in angiography, the imaging of contrast-enhanced blood vessels. Also fluoroscopy is used in specialized investigation like HSG, Barium series, etc. This is a demanding imaging task, requiring high contrast and sharp edge definition with low noise. Typically, much higher detector doses of around 100 to 300 µGy/min are used. Images were traditionally recorded using photographic film, but this has now been largely replaced by digital fluorography. Throughout the text of this manual, the term 'fluorography' refers to digital fluorography.

Fluoroscopy is the leading contributor of exposure to the US population from medical imaging. In 1995, the Food and Drug Administration (FDA) issued an advisory cautioning against the excessive use of high dose rate (HDR) fluoroscopy. There have been several documented cases of patients receiving burns from these units. It is therefore important to evaluate, on an ongoing basis, both the quality of the fluoroscopic images and the exposure output of the fluoroscopic system.

Fluoroscopic systems are part of the core imaging systems in the radiology department. Because they are used for many critical examination types such as interventional radiography and angiography, these relatively fragile systems should receive a great deal of attention in any complete quality assurance program. In many instances it would be appropriate to enlist the cooperation of the technologists who use the fluoroscopic rooms in the department as an integral part of the QC program.

The basic components of fluoroscopic and fluorography imaging units are:

- An X-ray tube and generator, which are capable of producing a stable X-ray output over long exposure times;
- A detector, capable of dynamic imaging, which is mounted opposite the X-ray tube;
- Digital image processing and storage facilities;
- A display system, for viewing real-time or recorded image sequences.

The specification of each component of the imaging system depends on the clinical tasks for which it will be used. There are three broad categories of fluoroscopic and fluorographic imaging equipment. These are described in the following subsections, along with some of their clinical applications.

1. For fluoroscopic X-ray units:

   Tabletop exposure rates.

   Centering alignment.

   Collimation.

   kVp accuracy and reproducibility.

   mA accuracy and reproducibility.

Exposure time accuracy and reproducibility.
Reproducibility of X-ray output.
Focal spot size consistency.
Half-value layer.
Representative entrance skin exposures.

2. For image-intensified systems:
Resolution.
Focusing.
Distortion.
Glare.
Low contrast performance.
Physical alignment of camera and collimating lens.

The goal of radiographic imaging is to demonstrate patient anatomy and pathology well enough to enable reliable, accurate diagnosis or intervention. If the balance between dose and image quality is to be optimised, suitable measures of image quality must first be defined.

Image Quality Characteristics

The fundamental characteristics that define image quality are described below:

Contrast

This is essentially the difference in signal intensity on imaging objects that have different attenuation coefficients. The greater the contrast between neighbouring structures, the more readily they can be distinguished. When the primary beam interacts with the patient, some of the X-ray photons are absorbed or scattered, and some pass through the patient to reach the detector and photoelectric absorption occurs.

Preferentially, materials with higher atomic numbers are the most important interaction process for diagnostic X-ray imaging. The probability of Compton scattering depends on electron density. Hence, it also contributes to image contrast.

However, those scattered photons that reach the detector produce a uniform increase in signal intensity across the image, and this has a detrimental effect on contrast.

There are three main sources of noise in a fluoroscopic or fluorographic imaging system. The first is quantum noise, caused by the random nature of the interactions involved in the production and detection of the X-rays. Since X-ray detection follows Poisson statistics, the signal-to-noise ratio can be improved by increasing the X-ray exposure. The second is noise arising from the structure of the detector itself, for example, the 'graininess' of the phosphor screens in an image intensifier. The third is electronic noise, which affects applied voltages in the detector, as well as the readout circuitry.

Resolution

In a digital imaging system, resolution is limited by the pixel size, inherent structure of the detector, and by processes such as scattering of the information carriers within it. Practical image resolution is also limited by geometric unsharpness; the X-ray focal spot has a finite size, and this causes a penumbra at the edges of imaged objects. Another factor affecting the resolution of medical images is motion unsharpness. This can be minimized by asking the patient to keep still and, where relevant, to hold their breath during image acquisition. In coronary imaging, motion unsharpness due to the beating of the heart is minimized by using pulsed imaging, with a rapid frame rate and short pulses.

Contrast Detail Tests

Subjective measures of low contrast detect ability can be made using standard or custom-built phantoms, and viewing the images by eye. The simplest phantoms contain fixed details of varying size and contrast. Some of the best known are the "Leeds" test objects developed by Hay *et al,* (1985) and currently marketed by Leeds Test Objects Limited (Boroughbridge, UK).

Figure below shows a radiographic image of the Leeds "TO.10" test object. This contains twelve rows of attenuating discs. Each row comprises discs of a different diameter, and the contrast varies from left to right, along each row. The observer views the image under a set of standard conditions, and counts the number of details visible in each row. The results are then compared with tabulated data, relating the number of details seen to threshold contrast, for given X-ray beam quality.

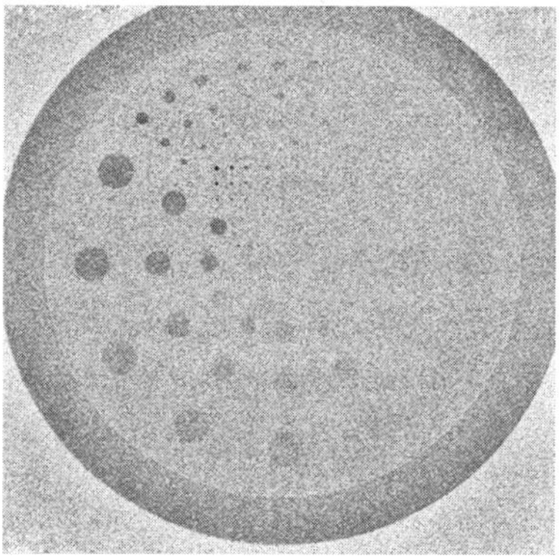

The tests are quick and easy to perform. They can be reliably used to detect large changes in system performance, and to rank systems according to their contrast and noise characteristics (Cohen *et al*, 1984; Marshall *et al*, 1992; Tapiovaara and Sandborg, 2004). However, they have a limited accuracy and reproducibility in identifying absolute threshold contrast, since they depend on the observer's subjective visualization threshold. This leads to inevitable variation between even the most experienced observers, and between viewing sessions, especially if they are separated by long time intervals.

Daily

Daily measurements of fluoroscopic systems are not necessary except under special circumstances. For example, if the radiologists are complaining of intermittent problems relating to resolution or noise, daily measurements for a short period may help isolate the nature of the problem. Suitable phantoms for daily evaluation of fluoroscopic image quality and system performance are available commercially.

Monthly or More Frequently if Indicated

System Function

A periodic check of the fluoroscopic system by the technologists who use the room on a daily basis is appropriate. Evaluation of spatial resolution and contrast resolution using a simple phantom (consisting of an attenuator, a wire mesh phantom, and a step-wedge) are important. Problems that can arise with the fluoroscopic system between the evaluations by the medical physicist may be identified during these periodic audits. The operator may track kV and mA required to produce an acceptable image as an index of system stability. The step-wedge may also be used as a daily check on monitor brightness and contrast settings.

Fluoroscopic Mode

Tested annually or more frequently, if indicated.

Typical Exposure Rates

The entrance exposure rate including backscatter for a "typical" patient should be evaluated at least annually. In some regulatory environments, more frequent (i.e. quarterly or monthly) evaluation may be required. This measurement requires the system to be set up in the same geometric configuration as it is used for typical patient examinations, using automatic brightness control mode. This usually involves placing thicknesses of PMMA (polymethyl-methacrylate or "acrylic") or another tissue-mimicking attenuator (10, 20, and 30 cm thicknesses are recommended) in the beam, and measuring the exposure between the X-ray tube and entrance of the PMMA. The Automatic Brightness Control (ABC) system should be activated, and operated in a typical clinical mode. The determination should be made in all available magnification modes. A radio transparent dosimeter is required for these measurements to avoid interference with the ABC system. If a free-in-air measurement is desired, a phantom material other than PMMA is required unless the geometry of the measurement can be altered to accommodate the necessary air gap.

Maximum Exposure Rates

The maximum patient exposure rate should be evaluated without backscatter; a PMMA scattering phantom should not be used. The maximum exposure rate should be determined by placing a sheet of lead over the input of the image intensifier, which causes the ABC circuitry to produce a maximum exposure rate. The image on the monitor should be blank, assuring that the ABC is driving the kV and mA to their maximum values. The exposure rate should be measured at the tabletop for under-table X-ray tube systems. If it is possible to adjust the distance between the X-ray focal spot and tabletop, this distance should be minimized. Image quality in fluoroscopy should be determined for two characteristics of the system, spatial resolution and contrast resolution.

Spatial Resolution

Spatial resolution of the system should be determined by tapping a line pair phantom to the center of the front surface of the image intensifier. The line pairs can be positioned 45 degrees with respect to the video scan lines and grid lines. Typically, a line pair phantom with the range of 0.7 line pairs per mm (c/mm) to 5 c/mm is used. With a copper plate (0.8 to 1.2 mm thick) placed in the beam at the collimator, the line pair corresponding to the highest spatial frequency that is visible under ABC-controlled fluoroscopy should be recorded. Both theoretical and achievable measured spatial resolution values have been published. It is important that the same individual be responsible for this test from time to time, to reduce the degree of subjective error. If multiple television monitors exist, the one used most by the radiologist during fluoroscopic studies should be used to make the measurement. Other monitors may be tested as well to identify monitor problems.

Contrast Resolution

Contrast resolution is determined by viewing a phantom containing various objects that span a range of subtle contrasts. The preferred phantoms for determining fluoroscopic contrast resolution are either the University of Alabama at Birmingham (UAB) phantom or the Leeds phantom. These phantoms consist of metal blocks or plates with holes of different depths bored into them. The systems have been calibrated at various kVs. The visual observation is made, and the kV recorded. With the calibration information, the absolute contrast resolution can be determined. A fluoroscopic system in good repair should resolve 11 mm discs at a contrast level <2%.

Radiographic Mode

Tested annually or more frequently, if indicated.

Kilovoltage Calibration

In fluoroscopy, the kV may be continuously changing as a result of the automatic brightness control. For most systems, there is a very little need to know whether the kV is accurate or not, since this knowledge will affect neither the image quality nor the dose to the patient in a direct sense. The easiest way to determine fluoroscopic kV is to use a non-invasive kV meter. These devices are commercially available, and, if carefully selected, simple to operate. The kV meter is placed in the fluoroscopic beam, and the kV is read out, kV indicators should be accurate to ±10%.

Radiation Quality (HVL)

The fluoroscopic circuitry in the X-ray generator is different from the radiographic circuitry, so radiographic beam quality results do not apply to the fluoroscopy capabilities of the unit. For fluoroscopic systems with manual kV control override, the preferred method for determining the HVL is to set the kV, and determine the HVL just as one would for a radiographic unit, measuring exposure rate instead of exposure. When a manual kV setting is not available on the fluoroscopic system, the HVL will have to be measured in ABC mode. To accomplish this, the field of view is minimized, and the exposure probe is placed as far away from the X-ray tube as possible. Several 1 mm sheets of aluminium are placed between the probe and the image intensifier. The sheets need to be big enough to span the minimized field of view and there needs to be enough of them to drive the kV to at least 80 kVp. The exposure rate is measured, and a single sheet of aluminium is removed from the stack behind the chamber and placed in front of the chamber midway between the X-ray tube and probe. Again, the exposure rate is measured, and the next filter is moved, and so on. This procedure keeps the same amount of aluminium in the beam for each measurement while varying the filtration in front of the probe. The ABC should be holding a constant mA and kV. In practice, knowing the HVL without knowing the kV is not that valuable, and so the kV reported by the fluoroscopic kV indicator on the system should be recorded. If the X-ray system does not have a kV indicator, there is no value in determining the HVL other than to assure compliance with state regulations.

X-ray anti-scatter grid: The grid can become dented or positioned incorrectly in the system with clinical usage. If possible, the X-ray grid should be removed from the system and radiographed using a detail screen film system.

Collimation

Confinement of the X-ray field to the image receptor (in both fluoroscopic and radiographic modes) should be verified.

Spot-Film Collimation

In radiographic mode the central ray of the X-ray beam should be aligned with the center of the image receptor, when placed in the Bucky, to prevent image cut-off and to avoid radiating tissues unnecessarily. Federal regulations currently mandate the edges of the X-ray fields and corresponding image receptor edges should agree to within ±3% of the SID. Tests should be performed at least annually or as often as necessary to maintain correct alignment. Further, the sum total of the misalignment in the X and Y dimensions should be less than 4% of the SID. Tests should be performed for enough image receptor formats to test each collimator blade position available.

Fluoroscopic Collimation

In fluoroscopic mode the central ray of the X-ray beam should be aligned with the center of the video image to prevent image cut-off and to avoid radiating tissues unnecessarily. Federal regulations currently mandate that the edges of the X-ray fields and corresponding image receptor edges should agree to within ±2% of the SID. Tests should be performed in all II magnification modes. Older systems usually require more frequent evaluation (*see* section 1).

Image Intensifier Input Exposure Rate (IIIER)

The IIIER, which is set by the service engineer during calibration of the system, has a direct effect on the entrance exposure rate to the patient. When the IIIER is set properly, the compromise between image noise and patient dose is such that the diagnostic quality is delivered at the lowest possible radiation dose. A proper IIIER setting also ensures that the typical patient entrance exposures will be reduced to the minimum exposure appropriate for the patient's size. With standard aluminium filtration added to the X-ray beam, IIIER values in the range of 1.5 to 2.5 μR per fluoroscopic video frame are typically set.

The measurement is made with the machine set up in its typical clinical geometry and the ionization chamber between the grid and the entrance plane of the image intensifier using the ABC mode. An attenuator, thick enough to drive the kV to 75 to 85 kVp is placed on the tabletop for each measurement. IIIERs' should be measured as a function of the following variables:

- Each magnification mode of the image intensifier
- Each IIIER setting the machine provides
- Each pulsed fluoroscopy frame rate

In addition to the above variables, most units have multiple modes of operation.

IIIERs' for all the following modes of operation that are available on the machine should be checked:

- Continuous fluoroscopy (analog, digital)
- Pulsed fluoroscopy (analog, digital)
- Any "high level" fluoroscopy mode
- Setup test exposure mode

The shape of the ionization chamber or design of the imaging system may not allow the medical physicist to place the ionization chamber at the entrance plane of the image intensifier behind the grid. In this case, the machine can be set up in its clinically used geometry and operated in the ABC mode with the appropriate phantom in place to determine the clinical kV, mA, and pulse width for the mode of operation. After recording these technique factors, the image intensifier can be moved to its maximum distance from the focal spot. The ionization chamber is placed "free-in-air" in the X-ray beam at the distance where the entrance plane of the image intensifier was located during the determination of clinical technique factors. The machine is placed in the manual mode which allows the operator to set the previously determined clinical technique factors. The exposure is recorded and corrected for the attenuation factor of the grid to determine the IIIER.

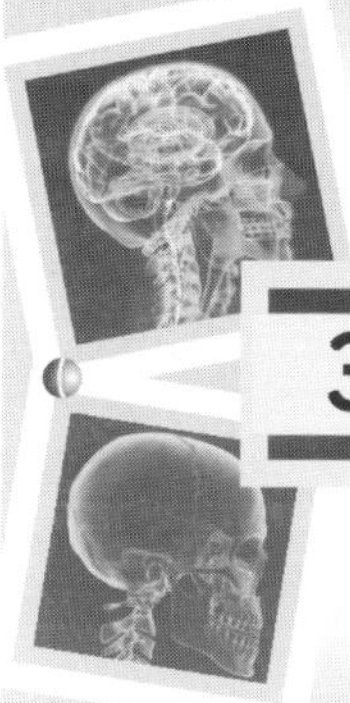

3 Quality Control in CT Scan System

Bushra Khan, Sumeet Bhargava, Satish K Bhargava

With its introduction in 1972, computed tomography (CT) revolutionized radiology. From initial scan time of several minutes for a single slice from a conventional (axial) CT, scan time have been reduced to just seconds for full volume acquisitions using helical or "spiral" CT and slip ring technology and to subsecond acquisitions for ultrafast electron beam CT scanners. Great improvements in image quality have also been realized through faster and more efficient detectors. Resurgence in CT has been recently realized with the rapid acceptance of multiple row or "multislice" CT scanners. CT scanners in clinical use today are generally either of the third-generation type (both the X-ray source and detectors rotate together) or the fourth-generation type (the X-ray source rotates around the patient while the detectors remain fixed). Helical CT units are available in both third- and fourth-generation designs while most modern multislice CT units are third generation designs.

Many of the QA tests for conventional scanners (or helical and multislice units operating in the axial mode) can now be performed using testing phantoms and protocols designed by the manufacturers. One must be careful utilizing CT phantoms produced in the 1970s. Because of the improvement in CT image quality, these early phantoms may not provide the means for testing the imaging limits of present CT scanners. The results of all QA tests should be compared to any manufacturer's limiting values and to the results of acceptance testing.

Daily

CT Number, Accuracy of Water, Image Noise, Image Uniformity, and Artifacts. These tests are combined since they are all obtained from the same CT phantom scans. They are also the most critical tests to be performed on a CT scanner, since they are sensitive to a wide range of CT scanner problems. This test involves imaging a water-filled (or uniform, water equivalent) phantom and using the statistics function of the CT scanner to determine the average CT number and standard deviation of the image noise in an ROI in the image. The image is also inspected for any nonuniformities or artifacts. The test for nonuniformities may also be performed quantitatively by obtaining average CT numbers over different areas of the image, e.g. central and four outer areas. Artifacts include the presence of "ring artifacts" which can be caused by miscalibration of the detectors in a third generation CT scanner or extra-focal radiation from the tube of a fourth generation scanner. Nonuniformities include shading or variations in the CT number over different parts of the phantom image. Examples are variations from one side of the phantom to the other and from the central to outer areas of the phantom. These tests should be performed daily using at least one common technique setting with a "head sized" phantom, typically about 20 cm in diameter . Analysis is simple and can be performed by the technologist. The average CT number and standard deviation of the noise should be obtained for a central region larger than $10 \times 10\ cm^2$. The size of the ROI used should be standardized for the QA tests. The image should be inspected visually for image nonuniformities and artifacts using a suitable window level and width. To properly visualize nonuniformities and artifacts, the window width should be relatively narrow, e.g. 50 to 100 Hounsfield units (HU). Use of excessively narrow window widths may enhance clinically insignificant artifacts. Significant artifacts or changes in mean CT number or standard deviation may be indicative of a malfunctioning system.

Semiannually or More Frequently, If Indicated

More complete versions of the above tests should be performed on a monthly to semi-annual basis, depending upon the available resources. In these tests images should be obtained using at least two different phantom sizes (e.g. head, body). Images should be obtained at all slice thicknesses used clinically. It is important that artifact scans be obtained at very thin slices and also in helical modes, if possible. If more than one kV and/or mA is used clinically, images should be obtained with those techniques. Images should also be obtained using different scan times and different reconstruction algorithms.

Imaged Slice Thickness (Slice Sensitivity Profile, SSP)

This test should be performed **monthly to semiannually** at all available slice thicknesses using an appropriate test phantom, such as aluminium or wire ramps for axial mode or a bead phantom for helical mode. The imaged slice thickness is usually taken as the full width at half maximum (FWHM) of the slice profile.

Dose Profile Width

This test should be performed **monthly to semiannually** at all available slice thicknesses. One quick method uses a packaged film, placed on the phantom surface during scans at the different slice thicknesses. The film is moved between scans so that a different area is exposed. The mAs technique is set to provide a maximum film density between 1.0 and 2.0 OD. Overexposure of the film must be avoided, since an incorrectly large value for the dose profile width would then be obtained. The developed film is then inspected under magnification to determine the dose profile width at the isocenter (correcting for geometric magnification). The measured dose profile widths should not significantly exceed the corresponding measured image slice thicknesses.

At acceptance, this test may also be performed on single and multi-slice "helical" (or "spiral") CT systems with the assistance of a CT engineer. "Ready-Pack" film is wrapped around a lead-lined, cylindrical object whose circumference is slightly smaller than the length of the film. The CT engineer removes the scanner cover allowing access to the pre-patient collimation. A strip of lead tape is used to block all but 1 cm of the fan beam, the opening being centered on the central ray. The phantom is placed at the scanner's isocenter and exposed using a variety of pitch settings.

The resulting patterns on the film allow for evaluation of table index relative to gantry rotation (actual pitch) as well as dose profile under dynamic conditions. Care should be taken to allow for magnification effects due to the finite radius of the cylinder. This test need only be performed at acceptance.

Slice Positioning Accuracy

QC comprises several tests that should be performed monthly to semiannually. These tests are for

- accuracy of the slice localization light(s),
- accuracy of slice positioning using prescriptions from the digital survey radiograph, and accuracy of the table motion with slice incrementation. In testing the accuracy of the slice localization lights, it is important to note the accuracy of each light that is used. In testing, the accuracy of the table motion, results should include the effects of reversal of the table motion.

CT Number Scale Accuracy and Stability

This test should be performed monthly to semiannually. A phantom containing a variety of materials with a wide range of CT numbers is scanned in axial mode using a set technique. The CT numbers of the materials are measured in the image and compared with standard values from the manufacturer and with previously measured values. Some typical materials used are polyethylene, water, PMMA, polycarbonate, nylon, polystyrene, and Teflon™. The measured values should remain relatively constant for a particular CT scanner. Large changes indicate malfunctions or calibration problems. The values obtained for identical materials can differ substantially for different CT scanners, due to differences in kV, filtration, detector absorption, and beam hardening corrections. When the CT number thus obtained is plotted against linear attenuation coefficient, a straight line should result with a correlation coefficient very close to 1.00, although the slope of this line will be equal to the CT constant used (typically 1000) divided by the linear attenuation coefficient for water at the effective beam energy in use. For a scanner that uses a CT constant of 1000 that is operated at 120 kVp with a hardened beam, the slope of the regression line should be 5200. Although this value will differ between scanners, it should remain constant (within ±5%) for a given system over time.

Spatial Resolution (Image Sharpness)

This test should be performed monthly to semiannually. In the axial mode, this test is most commonly performed by imaging phantoms containing suitable resolution objects in the x-y plane. These objects may be a series of rods of varying sizes that will image as dots, or a series of plates of varying sizes that will image as lines. Because there is more to visualize, the plate phantoms may sometimes indicate better resolution than rod phantoms. In call cases, the phantoms should be of high-contrast constructions with differences of typically 1000 HU between the rods or plates and surrounding material. The use of significantly lower contrast phantoms (e.g. 100 HU) is not recommended, though they could be used to give measurements related to the modulation transfer function (MTF). Older resolution phantoms whose smallest object sizes are greater than 0.5 mm are not suitable for resolution on present day CT scanners. Some CT scanners are capable of calculating resolution limits, MTFs, or point spread functions automatically by scanning a phantom containing a resolution phantom or thin wire. These results may be useful in providing alternative information regarding image sharpness. The thin-wire phantoms are sensitive to proper alignment along the z-axis. For helical CT the wire must have z-axis extension of at least the slice thickness plus twice the table feed per tube revolution. Measurements from a periodic rod or bar pattern may be more reproducible in clinical situations. The in-plane spatial resolution should be evaluated in the axial mode using both standard and high-resolution algorithms with a single slice thickness. Particularly with high-resolution algorithms, the pixel size in the standard scan field of view may limit the observed resolution, which may also be affected by the orientation and placement of the resolution pattern. In this case a smaller scan field of view may need to be imaged to demonstrate the true resolution capability of the CT scanner.

The in-plane spatial resolution in a helical scan at isocenter should be relatively independent of pitch and equivalent to that obtained from a conventional (axial) scan when all scan parameters are identical. However, if an appropriate phantom is available, the in-plane resolution for helical scans should be measured to verify equivalence. For reproducible results, the medical physicist should carefully evaluate any phantom used and select a pitch which limits the z-axis extension of the scan to avoid introducing artifacts. In clinical situations, both the in-plane and longitudinal resolution contribute to overall image sharpness and detail in helical scans. Unfortunately, there are a few, if any, commercial phantoms available to test longitudinal resolution for helical CT. A plastic "hole" phantom described by Polacin has been used with some success. Reconstruction software must be available to prepare multiplanar reformations (MPR) of the test object. If the appropriate software and a phantom are available, longitudinal resolution should be evaluated and monitored for several combinations of collimation and pitch. Reconstruction intervals should be chosen to be no more than 0.2 times the collimation.

Low-Contrast Detectability

This test should be performed quarterly to annually. It is important to perform this test in a way that minimizes the variations due to its subjectivity. Low contrast detectability phantoms should contain objects of less than 1% (10 HU) contrast, due to the improved imaging capabilities of modern CT scanners. The test phantom may contain objects of varying size and/or contrast. The phantom should first be scanned using typical clinical techniques, then using techniques higher and lower than those in clinical use. In the images, the smallest size objects that are perceivable at each contrast and technique level should be recorded. Visibility of large objects should improve with increasing technique. Small object visibility will also improve, but will ultimately be constrained by spatial resolution limitations.

To minimize errors due to the stochastic nature of the image, for each size and contrast several objects should be available for viewing. Because of the inherent subjectivity of this test, the performance of a particular scanner over time can probably be more precisely monitored using the image noise numbers. Because of the lack of commercial phantoms and general inexperience with three-dimensional (3-D) low-contrast measurements, helical low-contrast detectability in the longitudinal direction remains an issue to be resolved in the future.

Dosimetry of Axial Scans

These tests should be performed quarterly to annually. The method described by the FDA for dose evaluation is a measurement of the CTDI (CT Dose Index). We will refer to this measurement as the $CTDI_{FDA}$. This measurement requires the use of specified CTDI phantoms composed of PMMA with diameters of 16 cm and 32 cm and a cylindrical ion chamber with an active length of 14 cm. Exposure measurements are made by placing the chamber in holes near the surface of the phantoms and also at their centers. These measurements also require the use of lead filters to shorten the active length of the chamber when measuring slices thinner than 10 mm, since the exposure is only measured over a length of 14 times the nominal slice thickness. As a result, these measurements are cumbersome and time-consuming. Also the measurement results for slice thicknesses of 5 cm and below can quite misleading, since in such cases much of the single slice dose profile is excluded from the measurement. A much better CT Dose Index has been defined in a new standard from the IEC (International Electrotechnical Commission). In this measurement the exposure is measured over a 100 mm length for all slice thicknesses. As with the $CTDI_{FDA}$, this IEC measurement standard is performed with the ion chamber in holes near the surface and at the center of the phantoms and is then referred to as the $CTDI_{100}$. A weighted CTDI is also part of this standard and is obtained by adding together two-thirds of the surface $CTDI_{100}$ with one-third of the central $CTDI_{100}$.

$$CTDI_W = \frac{1}{3} CTDI_{center} + \frac{2}{3} CTDI_{periphery}$$

With this method, the requirement for the lead filters is eliminated and only a 10 cm chamber and phantoms are needed. Also, nearly all the single slice dose profile is detected in the measurement for all slice thicknesses. The $CTDI_{100}$ is very closely related to the MSAD (multiple slice average dose) for all measured slice thicknesses.

Manufacturers supply information on both $CTDI_{FDA}$ and $CTDI_{100}$ measurements for their scanners as a function of kVp, mAs, and slice thickness for surface and central ion chamber positions in both 16 cm and 32 cm diameter phantoms. The results obtained by testing of a particular scanner should correspond to the values provided by the manufacturer.

There are many pitfalls in the measurement of CT dose about which the reader should be warned. A specific flaw in the definition of $CTDI_{FDA}$ is the lack of a specified means of converting the exposure measurement into a dose figure. At CT energies the conversion factor (fmed) to convert exposure (R) to dose in soft tissue (rad) is approximately 0.94. However, most manufacturers use the fmed for PMMA of about 0.78 to calculate CTDI, and one must be aware of this usage. If the $CTDI_{FDA}$ is used in an attempt to calculate the dose to the patient (or to the embryo or fetus), the dose may be underestimated due to the lower fmed used and also due to the exclusion of significant parts of the single slice dose profile for thinner slices, as discussed above. The use of the $CTDI_{100}$, instead, mostly corrects these two problems. In the definition of $CTDI_{100}$ the fmed is explicitly given as that for air is 0.87. The measurement of surface dose by using a shorter cylindrical ion chamber on an imaging phantom will result in a substantial underestimate of the surface MSAD. Different CT scanners should not be compared by looking at only the central or surface CTDI or MSAD of a particular size phantom. Because of differences in pre-patient filters, different CT scanners have significant differences in the ratio of center to surface CTDI or MSAD. A robust method for routine measurement of the radiation dose from helical scans has not yet been described. However, the dosimetry for a helical scan at 1:1 pitch and 10 mm collimation is not appreciably different from that obtained with contiguous 10 mm axial slices. At this time, it is sufficient to verify performance using measurements of the $CTDI_{100}$ in axial modes only.

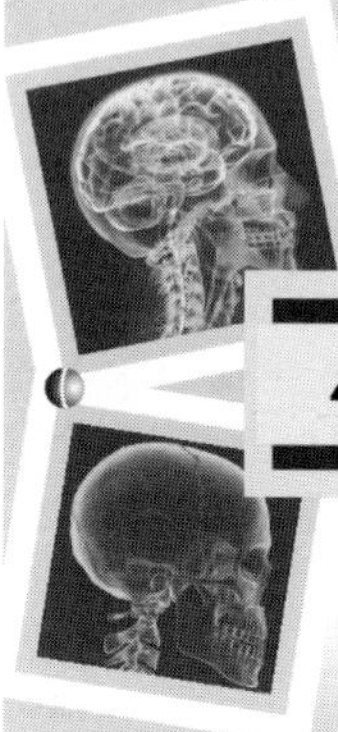

4 Quality Control in Ultrasound

Sumeet Bhargava, Bushra Khan, Satish K Bhargava

Equipment quality assurance is essentially performed every day during routine scanning by the sonographer and radiologist who should and can recognize major problems with the images and the equipment. Ensuring ultrasound image quality, however, requires implementation of a quality control program with periodic measurement of system performance to identify problems before serious malfunctions occur. Tissue-mimicking phantoms are required, having acoustic targets of various sizes and echogenic features embedded in a medium with uniform attenuation and the speed of sound characteristic of soft tissues. Various multipurpose phantoms are available to evaluate the clinical capabilities of the ultrasound system.

The system performance of a diagnostic ultrasound unit is described by several parameters: sensitivity and dynamic range, spatial resolution, contrast sensitivity, range/distance accuracy, dead zone thickness, and TGC operation. For Doppler studies, pulse repetition frequency, transducer angle estimates, and range gate stability are key issues. To ensure the performance, accuracy, and safety of ultrasound equipment, periodic quality control (QC) measurements are recommended. The American College of Radiology (ACR) has implemented an accreditation program that specifies recommended periodic quality control procedures for ultrasound equipment. The periodic QC testing frequency of ultrasound components should be adjusted to the probability of finding instabilities or maladjustment.

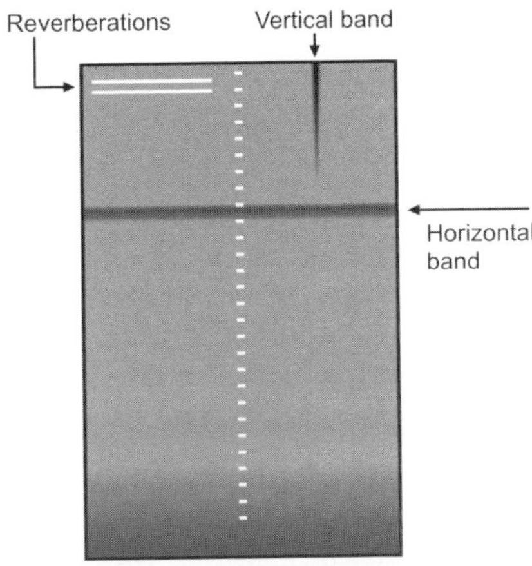

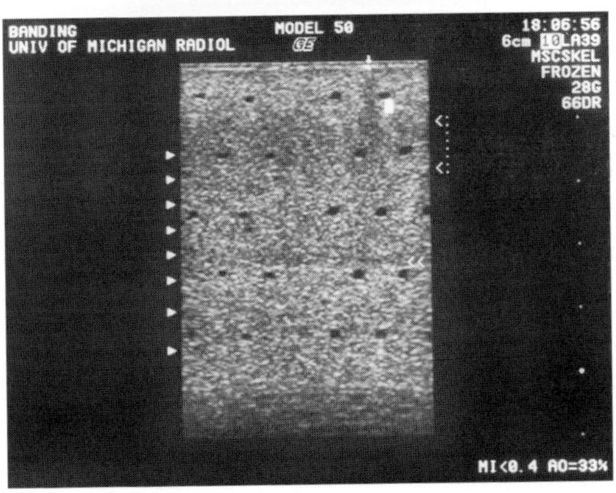

A generic phantom composed of three modules. The phantom gel filler has tissue-like attenuation of 0.5 to 0.7 (dB/cm)/MHz (higher attenuation provides a more challenging test) and low-contrast targets within a matrix of small scatterers to mimic tissue background. Small, high-contrast reflectors are positioned at known depths for measuring the axial and lateral spatial resolution, for assessing the accuracy of horizontal and vertical distance measurements, and for measuring the depth of the dead zone (the non-imaged area immediately adjacent to the transducer). Another module contains low-contrast, small diameter spheres (or cylinders) of 2 and 4 mm diameter uniformly spaced with depth, to measure elevational resolution (slice thickness) variation with depth. The third module is composed of a uniformly distributed scattering material for testing image uniformity and penetration depth.

Spatial resolution, contrast resolution, and distance accuracy are evaluated with one module.

Axial resolution is evaluated by the ability to resolve high-contrast targets separated by 2, 1, 0.5, and 0.25 mm at three different depths.

In an optimally functioning system, the axial resolution should be consistent with depth and improves with higher operational frequency.

Lateral resolution is evaluated by measuring the lateral spread of the high-contrast targets as a function of depth and transmits focus. Contrast resolution is evaluated with "gray-scale" objects of lower and higher attenuation than the tissue mimicking gel; more sophisticated phantoms have contrast resolution targets of varying contrast and size.

Contrast resolution should improve with increased transmit power. Dead zone depth is determined with the nearest high-contrast target (positioned at several depths from 0 to –1 cm) visible in the image.

Horizontal and vertical distance measurement accuracy is determined with the small high-contrast targets. Vertical targets (along the axial beam direction) should have higher precision and accuracy than the corresponding horizontal targets (lateral resolution), and all measurements should be within 5% of the known distance. Elevational resolution and partial volume effects are evaluated with the "sphere" module.

The ultrasound image of the spherical targets illustrates the effect of slice thickness variation with depth. With the introduction of 1.5-D transducer arrays as well as 3-D imaging capabilities, multiple transmit focal zones to reduce slice thickness at various depths are becoming important, as is the need to verify elevational resolution performance.

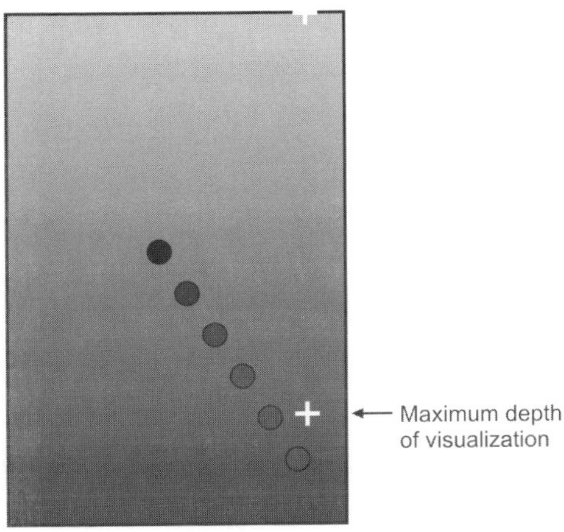

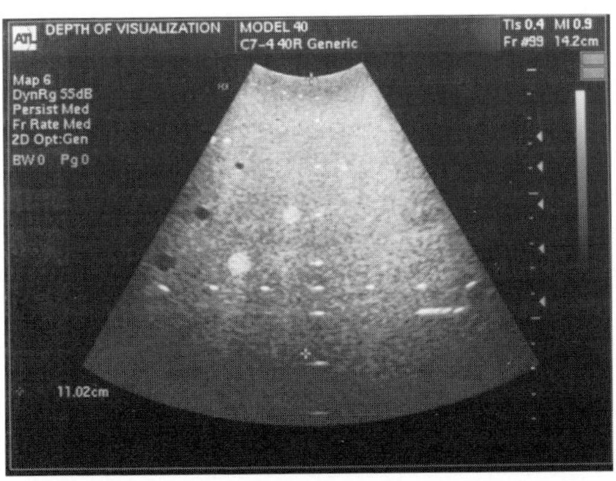

Uniformity and penetration depth is measured with the uniformity module. With a properly adjusted and operating ultrasound system, a uniform response is expected up to the penetration depth capabilities of the transducer array. Higher operational frequencies will display a lower penetration depth. Evidence of vertically directed shadowing for linear arrays or angular directed shadowing for phased arrays is an indication of malfunction of a particular transducer element or its associated circuitry. Horizontal variations indicate inadequate handling of transitions between focal zones when in the multifocal mode. These two problems are simulated in the figure of the uniformity module.

Recommended QC procedures for ACR accreditation are listed in the table below.

Recommended QC test for American College of Radiology (ACR) Accreditation Program

System sensitivity and/or penetration capability	Semiannually
Image uniformity	Semiannually
Photography and other hard copy	Semiannually
Low-contrast detectability (optional)	Semiannually
Assurance of electrical and mechanical safety	Semiannually
Horizontal and vertical distance accuracy	Semiannually
Transducers (of different scan format—ongoing basis)	At acceptance

Routine QC testing must occur regularly; a minimum requirement for accreditation is semiannually. The same tests must be performed during each testing period so that changes can be monitored over time and effective corrective action can be taken. Testing results, corrective action, and the effects of corrective action must be documented and maintained on site. Other equipment-related issues involve cleaning air filters, checking for loose or frayed cables, and checking handles, wheels, and wheel locks as part of the QC tests.

The most frequently reported source of performance instability of an ultrasound system is related to the recording of the images on film or the display on maladjusted video monitors. Drift of the ultrasound instrument settings or film camera settings, poor film processing conditions, and/or poor viewing conditions (for instance, portable ultrasound performed in a very bright patient room, causing inappropriately gain-adjusted images) can lead to sub-optimal images on both hardcopy (film) and softcopy (monitor). The analog contrast and brightness settings for the monitor and multiformat camera should be properly established during installation, and should not be routinely adjusted. Properly adjusting the video monitor brightness/ contrast knobs can be accomplished with image test patterns. A maximum window width and middle window level displays the minimum to the maximum gray-scale values, and allows the analog monitor contrast and brightness controls to be properly adjusted. Once adjusted, the analog knobs must be disabled so that image scaling is only applied using window level tuning from the scan converter memory. The image-recording (film) device is then adjusted to the same range of gray-scale values that appear on the soft copy device.

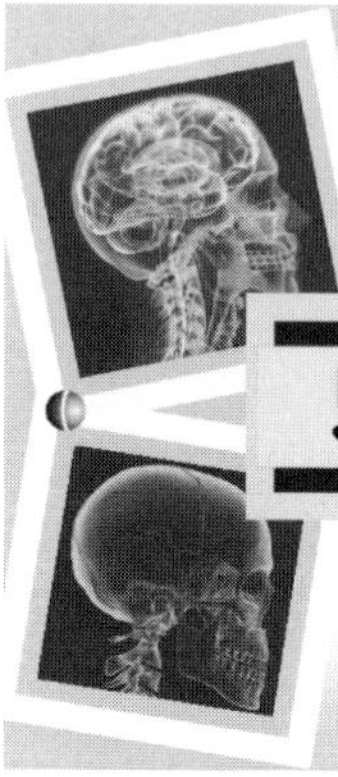

5 Quality Control in MRI

Sumeet Bhargava, Bushra Khan, Satish K Bhargava

The quality assurance for magnetic resonance imaging (MRI) requires phantom materials, phantom designs, and analysis procedures. Specific image parameters described in this manual are: Resonance frequency, signal-to-noise, image uniformity, spatial linearity, spatial resolution, slice thickness, slice position/separation, and phase related image artifacts. The primary considerations which dictate the choice of phantom materials for use in quality assurance phantoms are chemical and thermal stability, the absence of significant chemical shifts, appropriate T_1, T_2 and proton density values which are within the biological range. As coil loading is an important consideration while assessing signal-to-noise ratio, other considerations generally relate to convenience and practicality. Convenience by matching the T_1 of the material to an acceptable TR which does not require an exceedingly long scan time and practicality by not choosing a T_2 value shorter that some instruments can accommodate. Care should be taken to avoid the use of colored plastics or other container materials which possess significantly different magnetic susceptibility from the filler material.

For all measurements, scan conditions should be carefully recorded. Scan conditions should include: Pulse sequence and scan timing parameters (TE, TI, TR), flip angle, field-of-view (FOV) and matrix size, coil, phantom and phantom material, slice number and thickness, center-to-center spacing, number of acquisitions, rf power settings and any image processing which may have been used. All phantoms should be centered at the magnet isocenter unless otherwise specified.

Attributes given under should be carefully checked:

Daily

- Phantom setup
- Central frequency
- Transmitter gain/attenuation
- Geometric accuracy
- Spatial resolution
- Low-contrast detectability
- Image artifact assessment

Weekly

- Laser film QC
- Visual checklist
- Annual
- Physicist (or MRI scientist) performance evaluation

RESONANCE FREQUENCY

Methods of Measurement

Phantom

The phantom which is used most often for resonance frequency checks in a uniform signal producing cylinder and is the same phantom that is used for the signal-to-noise measurements. The phantom is positioned in the center of the magnet (with all gradient fields turned off) and the rf frequency is adjusted by controlling the rf synthesizer center frequency to achieve maximum signal. Some resistive systems may also allow adjustment of the magnet current to alter the magnetic field strength to achieve resonance.

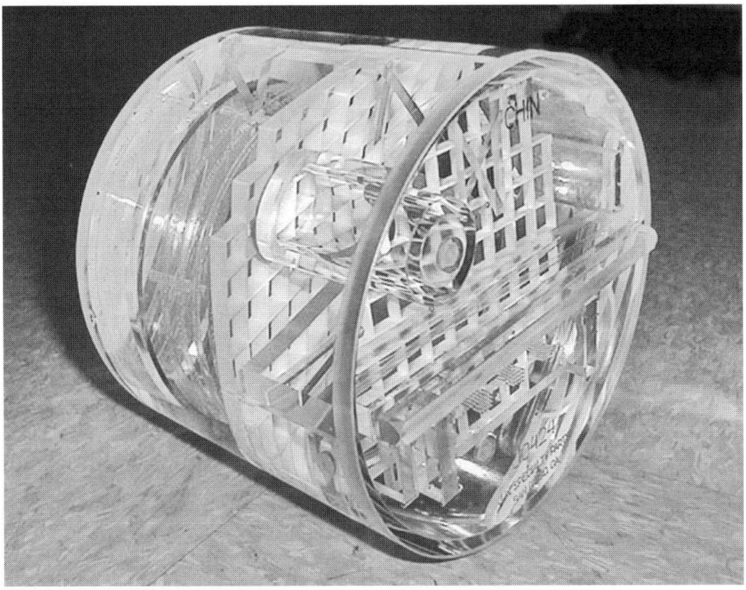

Most vendors will provide a specific user protocol for resonance frequency adjustment and some may be completely automated. Resonance frequency should be recorded daily for trend analysis.

Signal-to-Noise Ratio

Definition

The signal is defined as the mean pixel value within the region-of-interest minus any pixel offset. Noise is defined as the random variations in pixel intensity. Images with obvious artifacts are not suitable for signal-to-noise determinations.

Factors affecting signal-to-noise ratio

Factors contributing to variations in signal-to-noise ratio include: (i) general system calibration (resonance frequency, flip angles, etc.) (ii) gain, (iii) coil tuning, (iv) rf shielding, (v) coil loading, (vi) image processing, and (vii) scan parameters.

Methods of measurement

Phantom

The phantom should consist of a uniform signal producing material which has a minimum dimension in the image plane of at least 10 cm or 80% of the field-of-view, whichever is larger. For single slice measurements, the phantom should have a dimension in the direction of the slice selection which is at least twice the maximum slice thickness being used. For multislice acquisitions, the phantom length should be at least as long as the volume being imaged, plus two maximum slice thicknesses. The phantom may be either circular or rectangular in cross-section. When using large volume fluid-filled phantoms, it should be recognized that thermal and mechanically induced motions can introduce artifacts. The standard phantom specified here is to be filled with nonconducting material, and thus is not intended to simulate the clinical situation. The unloaded coil allows the evaluation of system noise which is the parameter of interest.

Image Uniformity

Definition

Image uniformity refers to the ability of the MR imaging system to produce a constant signal response throughout the scanned volume when the object being imaged has homogeneous MR characteristics.

Factors affecting image uniformity

Parameters contributing to the image nonuniformity include: (i) static-field in homogeneities, (ii) RF field non-uniformity, (iii) eddy currents, (iv) gradient pulse calibration, and (v) image processing.

Methods of measurement

Phantom

The characteristics of the phantom used for image uniformity evaluation are identical to the characteristics of the phantom used for signal-to-noise determination. To prevent rf penetration effects, the filler material should be nonconducting. Nonuniformities resulting from rf penetration effects may be evaluated by scanning a phantom which has been filled with a conductive solution such as normal saline. Due to partitioning in the body, penetration effects observed in a scan of a saline-filled phantom will not necessarily predict penetration effects which would be found in human scans.

Spatial Linearity

Definition

Spatial linearity is a term used to describe the degree of geometrical distortion present in images produced by any imaging system. Geometrical distortion can refer to either displacement of displayed points within an image relative to their known location, or improper scaling of the distance between points anywhere within the image.

Factors affecting spatial linearity

The primary factors which introduce geometrical distortion in NMR imaging are: (i) in homogeneity of the main magnetic field and; (ii) nonlinear magnetic field gradients.

Methods of measurement

Phantom

Variability is best observed over the largest field-of-view. The phantom to be used to measure spatial linearity should occupy at least 60% of the largest field-of-view and consist of a regular array of objects (holes, grooves, rods, or tubes) of known dimensions and spacing, and the phantom filled with signal producing material. The objects within the array should be of a size in which the location can be measured and spaced in a regular pattern (typically every 1–2 cm). The dimensional positioning error of the objects within the array, due to finite pixel size, should be < 10% of the linearity specification. The Figure provides an illustration of two possible patterns which could be used to evaluate spatial linearity.

The phantom used for spatial linearity should have a minimum dimension *(D)* in the image plane of at least 60% of the largest possible image field-of-view. The thickness of the phantom should be at least twice the maximum slice thickness for single-slice measurements and two slice

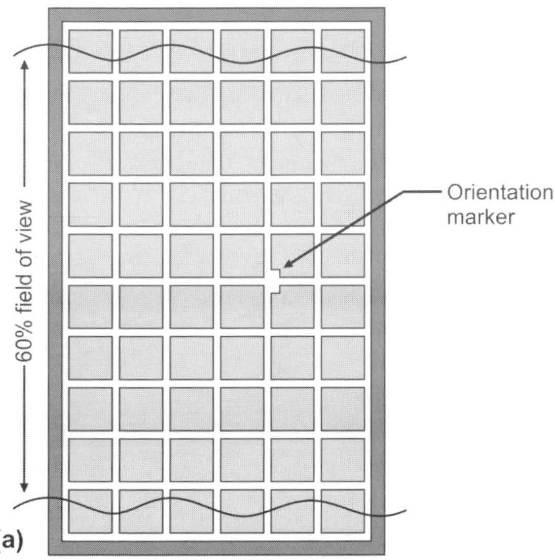

(a)

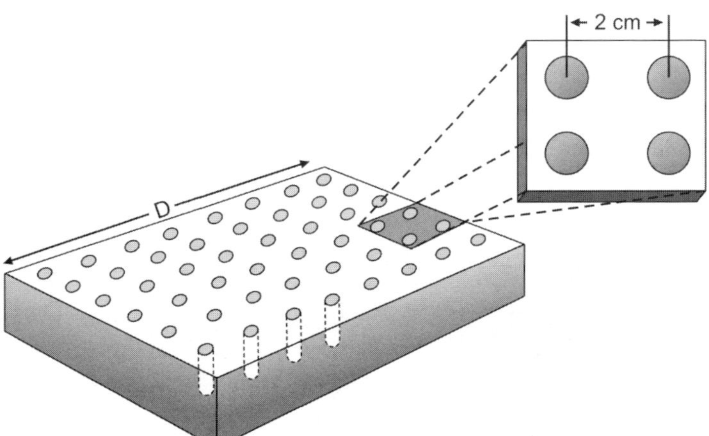

(b)

thicknesses, plus the image volume length for multislice measurements. Two possible phantom designs are (a) orthogonal grooves in an acrylic plate of (b) an orthogonal array of holes drilled in an acrylic plate. Orientation markers are recommended.

High-Contrast Spatial Resolution

Definition

High-contrast spatial resolution is a measure of the capacity of an imaging system to show separation of objects when there is no significant noise contribution. High-contrast spatial resolution for MRI systems is typically limited by

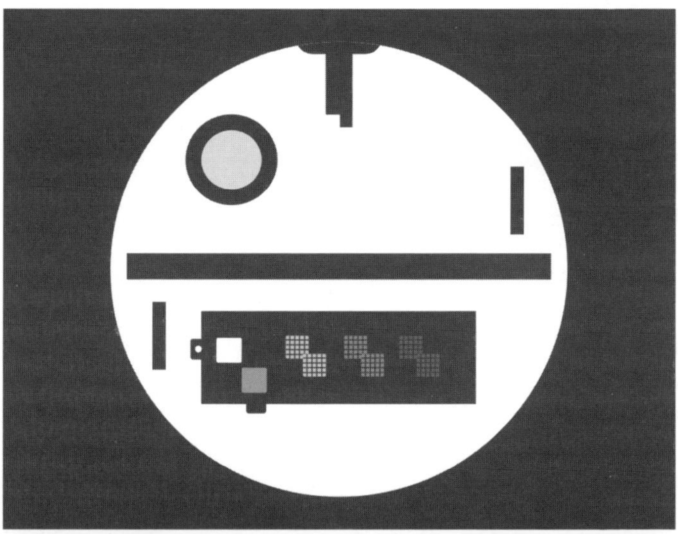

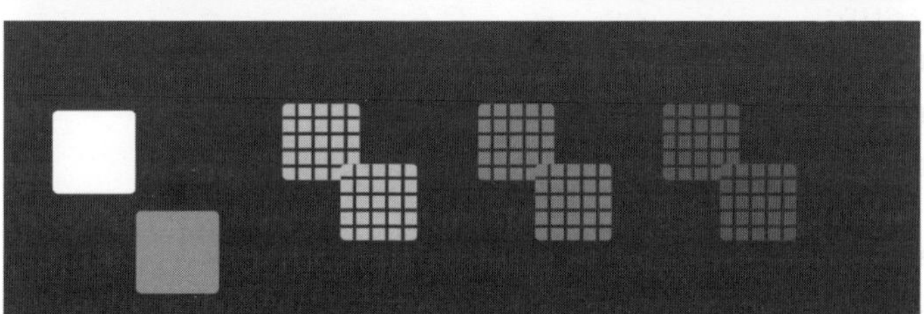

acquisition matrix pixel size (field-of-view divided by the sampling in x or y). The acquisition matrix pixel size should not be confused with the display matrix pixel size in which pixel interpolation or replication may have occurred. Traditionally, resolution has been quantified by the point spread function (PSF), line spread function (LSF), or modulation transfer function (MTF); however, these methods are not practical for routine quality assurance measurements on MRI systems. Therefore, a visual evaluation of test objects will be used.

Factors affecting resolution

Factors contributing to high-contrast resolution include: Field-of-view (determined by gradient strength and sampling period), acquisition matrix and reconstruction filters.

Methods of measurement

Phantom

Useful spatial resolution phantoms for visual evaluation may be composed of either bar patterns or hole (or rod) arrays. Array signal-producing elements may be either round or rectangular in cross-section. The patterns consist of alternating signal producing and non-signal producing areas set apart from each other by a width equal to the bar's or hole's width, i.e. center-to-center spacing is twice the diameter. Square bar patterns offer an advantage over round cross-section (hole) patterns in that the smallest resolvable array element can be related to resolution in terms of line-pairs per millimeter. If oblique planes are frequently used, consideration should be given to the inclusion of linearity measurements for oblique planes, as well as the orthogonal planes.

Analysis

Percent distortion is defined as distortion measurement may be performed between any two points within the field-of-view, provided that pixel-resolution is not a significant source of error. It is recommended that the true dimension be greater than 10 pixels. Preliminary considerations by the NEMA task group to specify image distortion have centered on the use of a cylindrical phantom in which several measured diameters are compared to the known diameter. Specification in terms of the maximum deviation (maximum–minimum) expressed as a percent of the known diameter is also under consideration. Spatial linearity measurements performed directly on the image processing unit will provide information about the MR imaging system alone. Measurements can also be performed upon filmed images and will provide combined performance information about the MR imager, as well as the video and filming systems. A typical phantom may consist of five signal producing elements and four spaces with element sizes of 5, 3, 2, 1.5, 1.25, 1.00, 0.75, and 0.50 mm, although additional increments may be used. The dimension in the slice selection direction (length) should be at least twice the slice thickness, i.e. 20 mm length for 10 mm slice thickness.

High-contrast resolution phantoms may be composed of either bar patterns or hole arrays. Bars or holes should have center-to-center spacings *(S)* equal to twice the hole diameter or bar dimension. The length *(L)* of the phantom should be at least twice the maximum slice thickness. Bars derived from grooves in an acrylic sheet may be preferred due to construction difficulties.

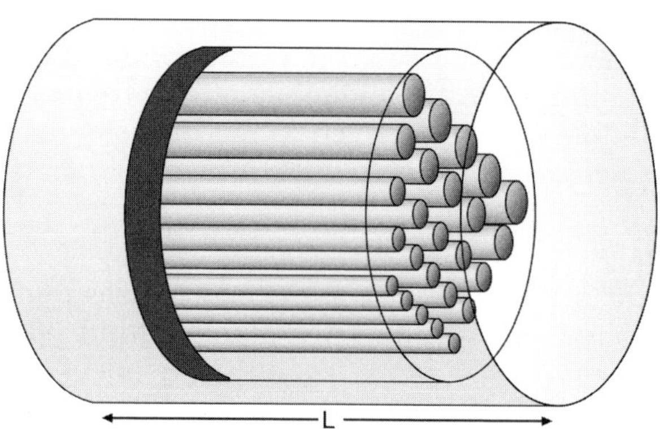

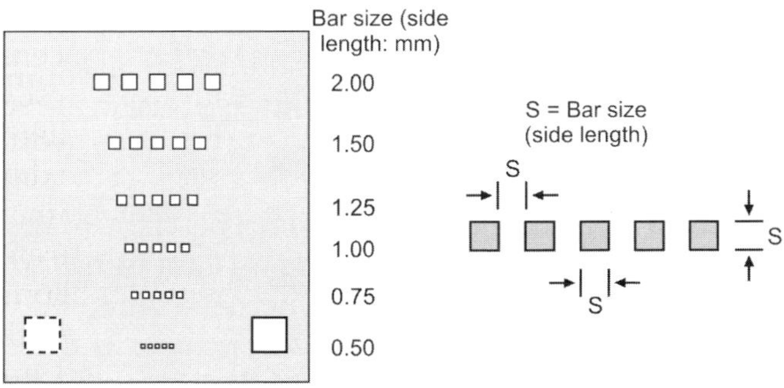

Slice Thickness

Definition

Slice thickness is defined as the full width at half-maximum (FWHM) of a slice profile. The full width at tenth maximum (FWTM) is an additional descriptor of the slice profile. The slice profile is defined as the response of the magnetic resonance imaging system to a point source as it moves through the plane of reconstruction at that point.

Factors affecting slice thickness

(i) Gradient field nonuniformity, (ii) rf field nonuniformity, (iii) nonuniform static magnetic field, (iv) noncoplanar slice selection pulses between excitation and readout, (v) TR/T_1 ratio, and (vi) rf pulse shape and stimulated echoes.

Methods of measurement

Phantoms

Several phantoms can be used to evaluate slice thickness, most of which utilize some variant of an inclined surface (plane, cone or spiral). A typical phantom is the crossed high signal ramps. High signal ramp (HSR) phantoms generally consist of opposing ramp pairs oriented at a fixed angle with respect to one another. The HSR's should be thin (ideally infinitesimally thin) in order to quantify the slice profile accurately. Because of the low signal in the image imposed by the small volume of signal-producing material in a thin ramp, averages of pixel values across the width of the ramp may be needed to generate a slice profile with an acceptable SNR. As thinner (<3 mm) slice thicknesses are evaluated, it is necessary to increase ramp angle and to decrease ramp thickness. In general, the thickness of a (90°) HSR oriented at 45° respect to the image plane should be <20% of the slice profile FWHM (i.e. 5 mm slice needs a 1 mm ramp) to get a measurement with <20% error. An alternative method which is particularly useful for evaluating thin slices is the use of the slice selection echo method. A standard selective 90° and 180° pulse sequence may be used together with a readout gradient oriented along the slice selection direction. The Fourier transform of the resulting echo gives a picture of the slice profile. The strength of the readout gradient is needed to translate the frequency axis to actual spatial dimensions.

A typical slice-thickness phantom consists of two crossed thin ramps. A ramp crossing angle of 90° yields an angle of 45° between the ramp and the image plane. Ramp thickness should typically be <20% of the slice thickness being evaluated. Phantom length *(L)* should be greater than twice the maximum slice thickness. An alignment rod passing between the two ramps defines the point where the two ramps cross. When the slice is properly aligned through the

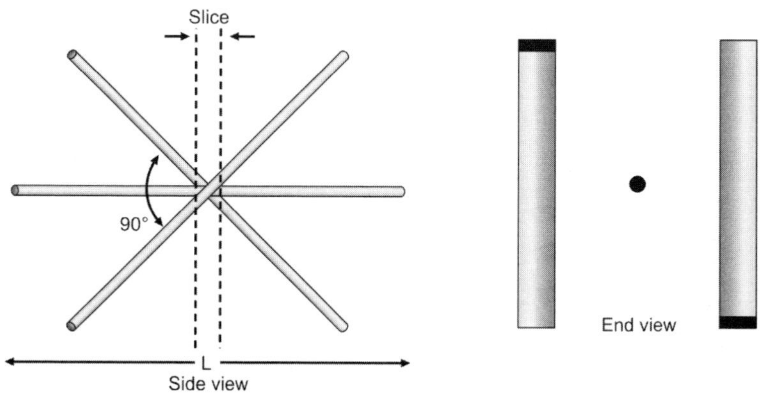

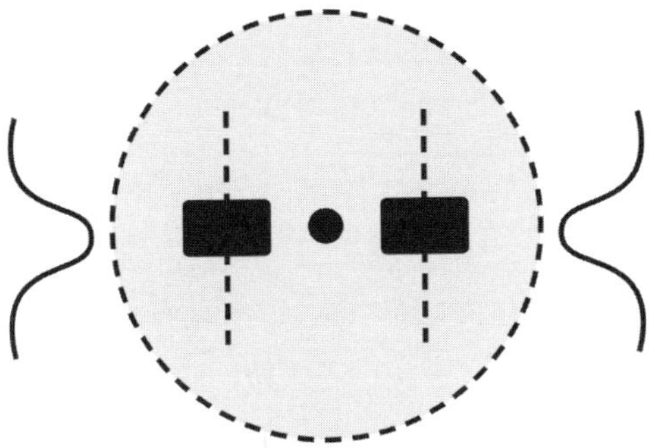

Scan image and signal profile

intersection of the ramps, the images of the ramps and rod image will all be aligned.

Slice Position/Separation

Definition

Slice position (offset) is the absolute location of the midpoint of the FWHM of the slice profile. Slice separation is the distance between any two slice positions. Slice locations are indicated by external positioning devices or by the selected inter-slice spacing.

Factors affecting slice position/separation

(i) Misalignment of positioning devices, (ii) gradient field nonuniformity, (iii) B_1 nonuniformity, (iv) noncoplanar slice selection pulses, and (v) static magnetic field.

Methods of measurement

Phantoms

In general, the same phantom used for slice thickness measurements may also be used for slice position/separation determinations, with the provision that the phantom contains reference pins and external scribed marks for orientation, centering, and reference to the external positioning devices. An inclined surface, with a known pitch, when imaged at different locations will produce images

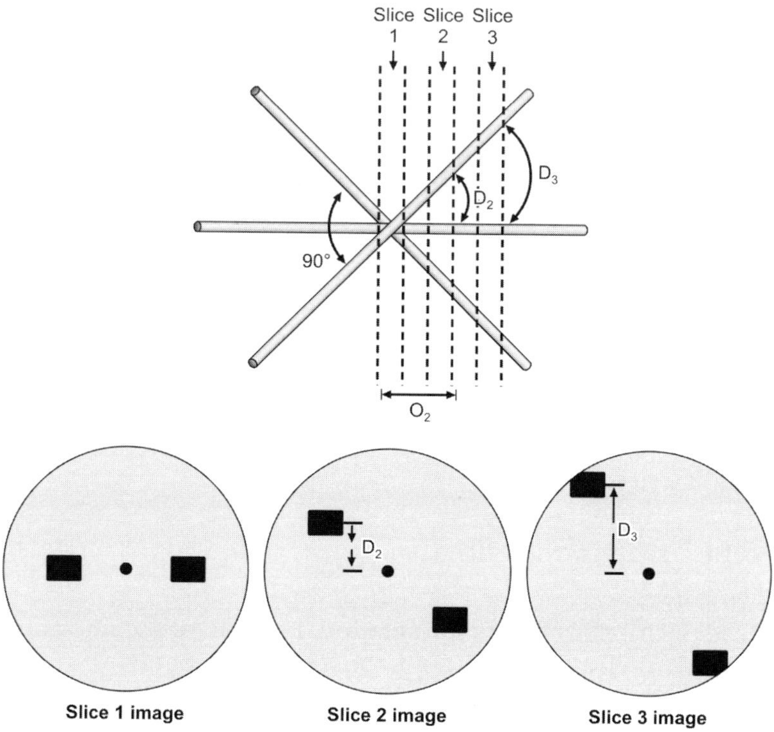

which will be displaced relative to a reference in direct proportion to the slice location and pitch of the surface.

Slice position (offset) and separation may be determined using a phantom similar to the slice-thickness phantom. Slices taken at different locations (slices 1–3) in a multi-slice sequence will produce images of the ramps which are progressively further from the alignment rod *(Di)*. The distance *D* is measured in the image and then related to the true slice location *(O)* from the isocenter.

Image Artifacts

Definition

Phase related errors are defined in terms of inappropriate (either increased or decreased) image signal at specified spatial locations. Generally, these artifacts are characterized by increased signal intensity in areas which are known to contain no signal producing material. Commonly called "ghosts", errors in the application of phase-encoding gradients for imaging and errors in both rf transmit and receive quadrature phase, result in unique ghost artifacts. A "dcoffset" error is defined here as high-intensity or low-intensity pixels at the center of the image matrix due to improper scaling of low-frequency components (typically DC) in the Fourier transformation of the NMR time-domain signal.

Factors affecting phase related artifacts

(i) Phase encoding gradient instability, (ii) quadrature phase maladjustment in the synthesis of slice selective RF pulses

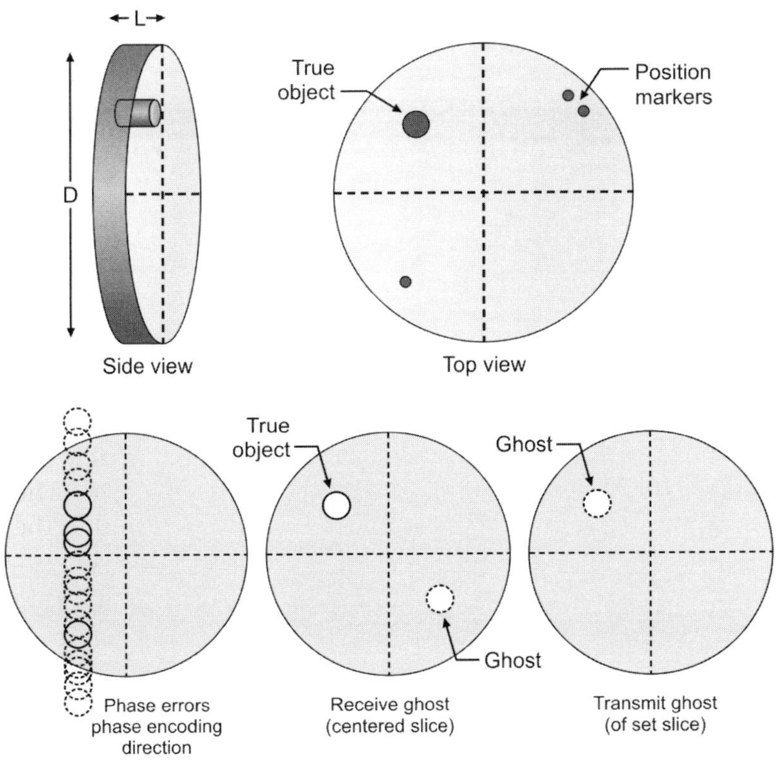

(transmit error), and (iii) improper quadrature phase decoding on receive.

Methods of measurement

Phantom

A typical phantom design is illustrated below. It consists of a single signal producing cylinder (2–5 cm) located at an asymmetric location, typically on the periphery of the field-of-view at a 45° orientation. The phantom thickness should be approximately twice the slice thickness being used. Orientation markers are particularly beneficial for this phantom.

A typical phantom for quadrature error detection consists of a single signal producing cylinder (labeled "true-object") located at an asymmetric location, e.g. at the periphery of the field-of-view at a 45° orientation. The size of the cylinder is not critical and may be as large as 2–5 cm in diameter. Marker sources are important for orientation information. Phantom diameter *(D)* should be at least 10 cm. Phantom thickness *(L)* should be at least two times the maximum slice thickness.

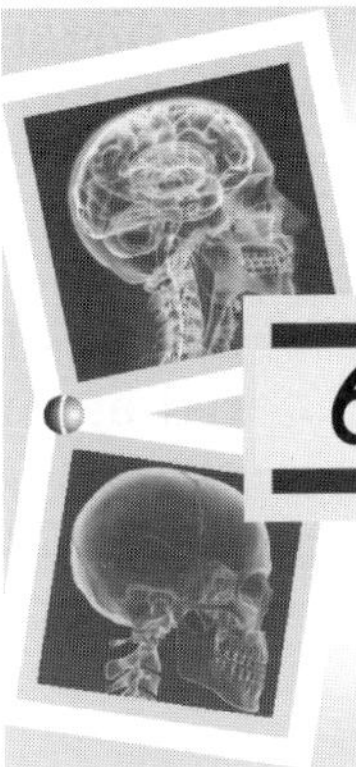

6 Quality Control in Nuclear Medicine

Bushra Khan, Satish K Bhargava, Sumeet Bhargava

INTRODUCTION

According to the Radiation Act (592/91), the responsible party shall implement planned and systematic measures to ensure that the radiation sources, accessories and associated equipment are in good condition and that the instructions and procedures concerning their use are appropriate.

Purpose and Scope

The purpose of this guidance is to introduce standards for quality control of nuclear medicine equipment and to give recommendations for a technical quality control programme. Technical quality control is an important part of the quality management of the nuclear medicine department. In this way it can be assured that the working order of nuclear medicine equipment is maintained within established requirements. For optimizing patient exposure during nuclear medicine examinations.

General Principles of Quality Control

A quality system is a system of organizational structures, procedures, processes and resources required in *quality management*. The quality system is described in quality documents that are arranged to be a uniform, constantly updated entity (a quality manual or similar). One means for quality management is *quality assurance* and *technical quality control* is part of it. There are also many other components of quality assurance and the main ones are mentioned below:

- Quality management
- Quality assurance
- Technical quality control
  1) acceptance testing
  2) regular quality control
- Activities administrated to patients
- Assessment of image quality
- Quality control of nuclear medicine
- Self assessment and clinical auditing

Technical quality control creates prerequisites for implementing the optimization principle. It is an integral part of the use of the equipment and the necessary resources should be seen as a part of the running costs.

In optimizing the dose from nuclear medicine examinations, the aim is to achieve an image quality adequate for making a diagnosis with a minimum radiation exposure possible.

The precision of the diagnosis that is achieved is influenced by many issues such as: Imaging, self-assessment and clinical auditing quality, technical, activities administered to patients, assessment of image quality, acceptance of regular quality, quality control of nuclear medicine, quality management assurance, testing quality control, control tests diagnostic reference levels, equipment, the object being imaged, the professional skills of the person performing an examination and the subjectivity of the person interpreting the image. Optimization requires in addition to technical quality control, an assessment of both the patient's radiation exposure and diagnostic image quality.

The patient's radiation exposure is linearly comparable to the activity of the radionuclide administered. This means that in optimization an adequate image quality is produced with the smallest possible activity. The activities used have to be compared regularly to the diagnostic reference levels established by the Radiation and Nuclear Safety Authority (STUK).

Phases and Content of Quality Control

The life cycle of an item of nuclear medicine equipment is established beginning from the intention to procure and ending at the disposal of the equipment, including tests performed during the working life cycle of the equipment. Quality control tests are conducted before taking the equipment into use (acceptance testing) and during clinical use of the equipment. According to the decree of the Ministry of Social Affairs and Health on the medical use of radiation, the functions of radiological equipment shall be tested in particular:

1. Before the equipment is commissioned (acceptance testing)
2. At specified intervals according to device-specific instructions (periodic testing)
3. Following significant repairs or servicing
4. When there cause to suspect a malfunction or a change in operation of an item of equipment

Quality Control Objectives and Test Groups

In this guide, quality control objectives of nuclear medicine equipment are divided into the following specific groups:

1. Gamma cameras
2. Coincidence cameras
3. PET cameras (PET: Positron Emission Tomography)
4. Combined imaging devices: SPECT-CT and PET-CT (SPECT: Single photon emission computed tomography; CT: Computed Tomography)

UNITS OF MEASURE

Système International d'Unités (SI) units shall be used in all reports of positron emission tomography performance measurements. Customary units such as milliCuries may be optionally reported as auxiliary values in parenthetical statements with the standard specifications for individual performance reports. The combined PET/CT scanner, introduced by Townsend and coworkers in 2000, overcomes this problem by providing precisely coregistered anatomical and functional images in a single multimodal imaging session. Commercial versions of this device, which first appeared in 2001, comprise separate PET and CT scanners with a common scanning bed, placed in tandem. After injection with a tracer and an appropriate uptake period, the patient is positioned on the bed and undergoes a spiral CT scan, followed immediately by a PET scan.

SPATIAL RESOLUTION

Introduction

The spatial resolution of a system represents its ability to distinguish between two points after image reconstruction. The measurement is performed by imaging point sources in air, and then reconstructing images with no smoothing or apodization. Although this does not represent the condition of imaging a subject in which tissue scatter and a limited number of acquired events require the use of a smooth reconstruction filter, the measured spatial resolution provides a bestcase comparison among scanners, indicating the highest achievable performance.

Purpose

The purpose of this measurement is to characterize the widths of the reconstructed image point spread functions (PSF) of compact radioactive sources. The width of the spread function is measured by its full width at half-maximum amplitude (FWHM) and full width at tenth-maximum amplitude (FWTM).

Method

For all systems, the spatial resolution shall be measured in the transverse slice in two directions (e.g. radially and tangentially). In addition, an axial resolution also shall be measured. The transverse field-of-view and image matrix size determine the pixel size in the transverse slice. In order to measure the width of the point spread function as accurately as can practically be achieved, its FWHM should span at least three pixels. The pixel size should be made no more than one-third of the expected FWHM in all three dimensions during reconstruction and should be indicated as a condition for the spatial resolution measurement.

Symbols

Resolution (RES)—The measurement of the size of the reconstructed image of a point source.

Resolution is specified as the **full width at half maximum** (FWHM) or **full width at tenth maximum** (FWTM) of the point source response.

Radionuclide

The radionuclide for this measurement shall be 18F, with an activity less than that at which either the percent dead-time losses exceed 5% or the random coincidence rate exceeds 5% of the total event rate.

Source Distribution

The point shall consist of a small quantity of concentrated activity inside a glass capillary with an inside diameter of 1 mm or less and an outside diameter of less than 2 mm. The axial extent of the activity in the capillary shall be less than 1 mm.

The sources shall be fixed parallel to the long axis of the tomograph and located at 6 points as follows:

- In the axial direction, along planes
  (1) at the center of the axial FOV, and

(2) one-fourth of the axial FOV from the center of the FOV.

- In the transverse direction the source shall be positioned
  (1) 1 cm vertically from the center (to represent the center of the FOV, but positioned to avoid any possible inconsistent results at the very center of the FOV),
  (2) at $x = 0$ and $y = 10$ cm, and
  (3) at $x = 10$ cm and $y = 0$.

Data Collection

Measurements shall be collected at all six positions specified above. At least one hundred thousand counts shall be acquired in each response function. Measurements can be taken with multiple sources. Finer sample size may be selected than typically used in clinical studies.

Data Processing

Reconstruction by filtered back projection with no smoothing or apodization shall be employed for all spatial resolution data.

Analysis

The spatial resolution (FWHM and FWTM) of the point source response function in all three directions shall be determined by forming one-dimensional response functions, along profiles through the image volume in three orthogonal directions, through the peak of the distribution. The width of the response functions in the two directions at right angles to the direction of measurement shall be approximately two times the FWHM.

Each FWHM (and FWTM) shall be determined by linear interpolation between adjacent pixels at half (or one-tenth) the maximum value of the response function. The maximum value shall be determined by a parabolic fit using the peak point and its two nearest neighboring points.

SCATTER FRACTION, COUNT LOSSES, AND RANDOMS MEASUREMENT

Introduction

The scattering of gamma rays emitted by the annihilation of positrons results in falsely located coincidence events. Variations in design and implementation cause positron emission tomographs to have different sensitivities to scattered radiation.

The measurements of count losses and random rates express the ability of a positron emission tomograph to measure highly radioactive sources with accuracy.

Purpose

The first purpose of this procedure is to measure the relative system sensitivity to scattered radiation. Scatter is expressed by the scatter fraction (SF) for the entire tomograph. The second purpose of this procedure is to measure the effects of system dead-time and the generation of random events at several levels of source activity.

The true event rate is the total coincident event rate minus the scattered event rate and minus the randoms event rate. The method of random estimation includes misplaced events as part of the randoms measurement. Furthermore, shifts in the energy peak may influence the results for the randoms, since it is assumed that the scatter fraction is constant as a function of count rate.

Method

The test phantom is a solid right circular cylinder composed of polyethylene with a specific gravity of 0.96 ±0.01, with an outside diameter of 203 ±3 mm (8"), and with an overall length of 700 ±5 mm. A 6.4 ±0.2 mm (0.25") hole is drilled parallel to the central axis of the cylinder, at a radial distance of 45 ±1 mm. For ease of fabrication and handling, the cylinder may consist of several segments that are assembled together during testing. However, in both design and assembly of the completed phantom, one must *insure a tight fit between adjacent segments*, as even very small gaps will allow narrow axial regions of scatter-free radiation.

The test phantom line source insert is a clear polyethylene or polyethylene-coated plastic tube at least 800 mm in length, with an inside diameter of 3.2 ±0.2 mm (1/8") and an outside diameter of 4.8 ±0.2 mm (3/16"). The central 700 ±5 mm of this tube will be filled with a known quantity of activity and threaded through the 6.4 mm hole in the test phantom.

To begin the test, a source of relatively high activity is placed in the field of view of the positron emission tomograph. Regular measurements are then taken while the activity in the phantom decays over several half-lives. A decrease in the ratio of the random event rate to the true event rate accompanies the activity decay, eventually falling to less than 1%. In addition, the efficiency of the system in processing coincident events improves as the activity decays, until count losses may be effectively neglected. Thus by waiting long enough one obtains a measurement of the coincidence count rate that is effectively free from both randoms and processing losses.

Extrapolating this true rate back to higher activity levels and comparing it to the measured rate, one may estimate count losses suffered by the system at higher activity levels. The accuracy of this technique depends critically on adequate statistics being gathered at sufficiently low levels of activity. This may require repeated measurements at the lower count rates.

Symbols

Scatter fraction(SF): A dimensionless ratio of scattered coincidence events to the sum of scattered and true coincidence events in a defined ROI of the scanner field-of-view.

Radionuclide

The radionuclide used for this measurement shall be 18F. The amount of radioactivity shall be great enough to allow the following two rates to be measured:

a. Rt, peak—peak true count rate

b. RNEC, peak—peak noise equivalent count rate

Recommendations for the initial activity required to meet these objectives will be supplied by the manufacturer.

The initial activity in the phantom shall be determined from the activity injected into the phantom as measured in a calibrated dose calibrator.

Source Distribution

The central 700 ±5 mm of the test phantom line source insert shall be filled with water mixed with the measured amount of radioactivity and sealed at both ends. This line source shall be inserted into the hole of the test phantom such that the region of activity coincides with the 70 cm length of the phantom. The test phantom with line source is mounted on the standard patient table supplied by the manufacturer and rotated such that the line source insert is positioned nearest to the patient bed (*see* Fig. 1). The phantom is centered in the transverse and axial fields-of-view to within 5 mm.

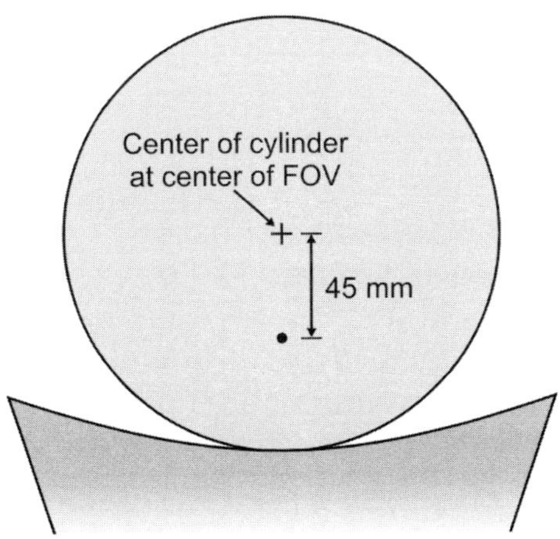

Fig. 1 Positioning of phantom

Data Collection

Data shall be acquired at intervals more frequent than half the radionuclide half-life (t½), until true events losses are less than 1.0%, and the random rates are less than 1.0% of true rates. The durations of the individual acquisitions, $T_{acq} - j$, shall be less than one-fourth of t½. Acquisitions shall be fully tomographic; therefore, rotating scanners must rotate to provide complete and uniform angular sampling for each acquisition. In the case of rotating scanners, the acquisition time $T_{acq} - j$ shall include the time required to rotate the detectors.

POSITIONING OF PHANTOM

It is essential to the accurate estimation of system dead-time losses that sufficient statistics be acquired with count loss rates and random rates both below 1.0% of true rates. Each acquisition should contain a minimum of 500,000 prompt counts. It is also important that the measurements around the peak count rate be done with sufficient frequency so that the peak rate can be accurately determined. Therefore, it is expected that manufacturers will recommend a protocol for their scanners that includes starting activity, acquisition time, and durations.

Data Processing

For tomographs with an axial field of view of 65 cm or less, sinograms shall be generated for each acquisition (j) of slice i. For tomographs with an axial field of view greater than 65 cm, sinograms shall be generated for each acquisition for slices within the central 65 cm. No corrections for variations in detector sensitivity or detector motions such as wobble, randoms, scatter, dead-time, or attenuation shall be applied to the measurements. Real-time subtraction of random events shall not be done.

The sinograms must contain the total acquired counts of the scanner without corrections; i.e., the sinograms must contain true, random, and scatter counts. Furthermore, scanners with the capacity for direct measurement of random rates may not use these measurements in the estimation of random count rates detailed below. Oblique sinograms are collapsed into a single sinogram for each respective slice (by single-slice rebinning) while conserving the number of counts in the sinogram.

Analysis

All pixels in each sinogram i of acquisition j located farther than 12 cm from the center of the phantom shall be set to zero. For each projection angle a within the sinogram, the location of the center of the line source response shall be determined by finding the pixel having the greatest value. Each projection shall be shifted so that the pixel containing the maximum value is aligned with the central pixel of the sinogram. After alignment, a sum projection shall be produced such that a pixel in the sum projection is the sum of the pixels in each angular projection having the same radial offset as the pixel in the sum projection.

Sensitivity

Sensitivity of a positron emission tomograph is expressed as the rate in counts per second that true coincidence events are detected for a given source strength. Since the emitted positrons annihilate and create a pair of gamma rays, a significant amount of material must surround the source to insure annihilation. This surrounding material also attenuates the created gamma rays, prohibiting a measurement without interfering attenuation. To arrive at an attenuation free measurement, successive measurements are made with a uniform line source surrounded by known absorbers. From these measurements, the sensitivity with no absorber can be extrapolated.

Purpose

The purpose of this procedure is to measure the sensitivity or ability of the scanner to detect positrons.

Method

The test equipment required for this measurement is the sensitivity phantom.

Symbols

Accumulated sleeve wall thickness (*X*): The combined thickness of the metal sleeve walls used in the sensitivity measurement.

Attenuation coefficient (*m*): A measure of the likelihood that a photon will undergo an interaction while travelling through a material, expressed in units of reciprocal distance (such as mm^{-1}).

Sensitivity (*S*): A measure of the rate at which coincidence events are detected in the presence of radioactive sources in the limit of low activity levels where count rate losses are negligible.

(a) *Si* – sensitivity of slice *i*

(b) S_{tot} – total system sensitivity

Radionuclide

The radionuclide employed for these measurements shall be 18F. The activity used shall be low enough so that the counting losses are less than one percent, and the random event rate is less than 5% of the true rate. The initial activity in the phantom shall be determined by measurement in a dose calibrator.

Source Distribution

A 700 ±5 mm portion of plastic tubing shall be filled with water, well mixed with a measured amount of radioactivity, and sealed at both ends. This activity, A_{cal} in MBq, and the time of the assay, T_{cal}, should be recorded. The phantom is suspended in the center of the transaxial field of view, aligned with the axis of the tomograph in such a way that any supporting mechanism is external to the field-of-view.

Data Collection

Data are collected for a period of time to ensure that at least 10,000 trues per slice are collected. Single slice rebinning shall be used to assign counts in oblique lines-of-response (LOR) to the image slice where the LOR crosses the scanner axis. The time of the measurement, T_1, is recorded along with the duration, T_{acq}, and the number of counts collected. In the case of scanners whose detectors must be moved to acquire a full tomographic data set, the acquisition time T_{acq} shall include the time required to move the detectors. The rate, R_1, *i*, in counts per second, shall be determined by dividing the counts collected in the slice by the duration. In succession, each of the four sleeves are added to the phantom and the measurement repeated, recording values for *Tj* and *Rj*, *i* for each measurement.

To assess the sensitivity at different radial positions, the process described in the preceding paragraph shall be repeated at 10 cm radial offset from the center of the transaxial field-of-view.

ACCURACY: CORRECTIONS FOR COUNT LOSSES AND RANDOMS

Introduction

To achieve quantitative measurements of source activity distributions under widely varying conditions, positron emission tomographs usually have a capability to compensate for dead time losses and random events. The accuracy of these corrections, particularly at the highest count rates encountered in clinical imaging, is reflected by the bias with which the tomograph reports counts. The following test uses a simple activity distribution and clearly is not representative of a wide variety of imaging conditions. However, such a test requires a considerable amount of time to perform and requires handling large amount of radioactivity.

Purpose

The purpose of this procedure is to measure the accuracy of corrections for dead-time losses and random event counts in images.

Method

The test phantom data, acquired for measurements of random rates and dead time losses, can also be used to measure the net error in count rate after correction for dead time losses and randoms subtraction.

The comparison is between the corrected true count rate and the expected count rate extrapolated from low count rate data. Errors from dead-time and randoms are assumed to be insignificant at low count rates. All corrections are to be applied.

Symbols

Relative count rate error (Dr): The difference between the expected count rate and the measured count rate, expressed as a percentage of the expected rate.

Radionuclide

The radionuclide used for this measurement shall be 18F. The amount of radioactivity shall be great enough to cause the true event rate to reach a 50% dead-time loss value and also to allow the following two rates to be measured:

(a) Rt, peak – peak true count rate

(b) RNEC, peak – peak noise equivalent count rate

Recommendations for the initial activity required to meet these objectives will be supplied by the manufacturer.

The initial activity in the phantom shall be determined from the activity injected into the phantom as measured in a calibrated dose calibrator.

Source Distribution

The central 700 ±5 mm of the test phantom line source insert shall be filled with water, well mixed with the measured amount of radioactivity, and sealed at both ends. This line source shall be inserted into the hole of the test phantom such that the region of activity coincides with 70 cm length of the phantom. The test phantom with line source is mounted on the standard patient table supplied by the manufacturer and rotated such that the line source insert is positioned nearest to the patient bed. The phantom is centered in the transverse and axial fields-of-view.

Data Collection

Data shall be acquired at intervals more frequent than half the radionuclide half-life (t½), until count loss rates of true events are less than 1.0% of the total, and the random rates are less than 1.0% of true rates. The durations of the individual acquisitions, T_{acq}, j, shall be less than one-fourth of t½. Acquisitions shall be fully tomographic; therefore, rotating scanners must rotate to provide complete and uniform angular sampling for each acquisition.

It is essential to the accurate estimation of system dead-time losses that sufficient statistics be acquired with count loss rates and random rates both below 1.0% of true rates. Each acquisition should contain a minimum of 500,000 prompt counts. Therefore, it is expected that manufacturers will recommend a protocol for their scanners that includes starting activity, acquisition times, and the duration.

Data Processing

For tomographs with an axial field of view of 65 cm or less, all slices shall be reconstructed. For tomographs with an axial field-of-view greater than 65 cm, only slices in the central 65 cm shall be reconstructed. Randoms and deadtime corrections shall be applied to the data. Images shall be reconstructed using the standard means and that method shall be reported.

Analysis

All analyses shall be performed on each reconstructed image *i*. The average activity A_{ave}, *j* for each acquisition *j* shall be calculated. The average effective activity concentration A_{eff}, *j* for each acquisition *j* shall be computed by dividing A_{ave}, *j* by the volume of the test phantom (22,000 cm^3).

IMAGE QUALITY, ACCURACY OF ATTENUATION AND SCATTER CORRECTIONS

Introduction

Because of the complex interplay of different aspects of system performance, it is desirable to be able to compare the image quality of different imaging systems for a standardized imaging situation that simulates a clinical imaging condition. Due to variations in the uptake of radiopharmaceuticals and in-patient sizes and shape, it is difficult to simulate clinical imaging conditions using a phantom. For these reasons, the results of a single phantom study can only give indications of image quality for that particular imaging situation.

Purpose

The purpose of this measurement is to produce images simulating those obtained in a total body imaging study with both hot and cold lesions. Spheres of different diameters are imaged in a simulated body phantom with non-uniform attenuation; activity is also present outside the scanner. Image contrast and signal-to-noise ratios for both hot and cold spheres are used as measures of image quality. In addition, the accuracy of the attenuation and scatter corrections is determined from this measurement.

Method

Symbols

Contrast (Qxxx): The contrast of a sphere in a warm background:

(a) QH – hot sphere contrast

(b) QC – cold sphere contrast

Background variability (Nxxx): Used as part of the image quality measurement:

- *Nj*—coefficient of variation for all ROIs of size *j* in the image volume.

Relative count error (DC): The difference between the expected and measured counts, expressed as a percentage:

- DC lung—relative error in lung insert

Standard deviation (SDxxx): Used as part of the background variability measurement:

- SD*j*—standard deviation for all ROIs of size *j* in the image volume

Radionuclide

The radionuclide for this measurement shall be 18F. The concentration of the background activity in the phantom shall be 5.3 kBq/cc (0.14 mCi/cc) within ±5% as calibrated at the start of imaging. This activity concentration corresponds to 370 MBq (10 mCi) per 70,000 cc, a typical injected dose for total body studies. If the manufacturer suggests a lower injected activity for total body imaging, a corresponding lower background activity concentration may be used for this study. The background activity concentration used and the manufacturer's recommended injected dose for total body imaging shall be reported. The cold lesions shall be filled with water containing no radioactivity. The hot lesions shall be filled with a concentration of *N* times that of the background, where *N* = 4 and 8. The line source of the test phantom shall be filled with 116 MBq (3.08 mCi). 18F to yield an effective activity "concentration" equal to the background activity concentration, if a lower background activity is used in the phantom, then a corresponding lower activity shall be used in the line source, as well.

Source Distribution

The imaging phantom consists of four parts:

(a) A body phantom of at least 180 mm interior length,

(b) Six fillable spheres with internal diameters of 10, 13, 17, 22, 28, and 37 mm with a wall thickness of less than or equal to 1 mm.

(c) To simulate the attenuation of lung, a cylindrical insert filled with a low atomic number material with an average density of 0.30 ±0.10 g/cc, 50 ±2 mm in outside diameter with a wall thickness less than 4 mm, that is centered inside the body phantom and that extends through the entire axial extent of the phantom; and

d. The test phantom (line source in solid polyethylene cylinder) used for the scatter fraction, and count losses.

The two largest spheres (28 mm and 37 mm) shall be filled with water for cold lesion imaging, and the four smallest spheres (10 mm, 13 mm, 17 mm, and 22 mm) with 18F for hot lesion imaging. The centers of the spheres shall be placed 68 mm from the body phantom endplate so that they are axially in the same transverse slice. The transverse positioning of the spheres shall be so that the centers of the spheres are positioned at a radius of 5.72 cm from the center of the phantom, Fig. 2. The 17 mm diameter sphere shall be positioned along the horizontal axis of the phantom.

The body phantom shall be filled with the background activity concentration and placed on the imaging table. The body phantom shall be positioned axially in the scanner so that the center of the spheres is at the middle slice of the scanner and positioned transaxially so that the center of the phantom is centered in the scanner. The phantom shall be aligned so that the plane through the centers of the spheres

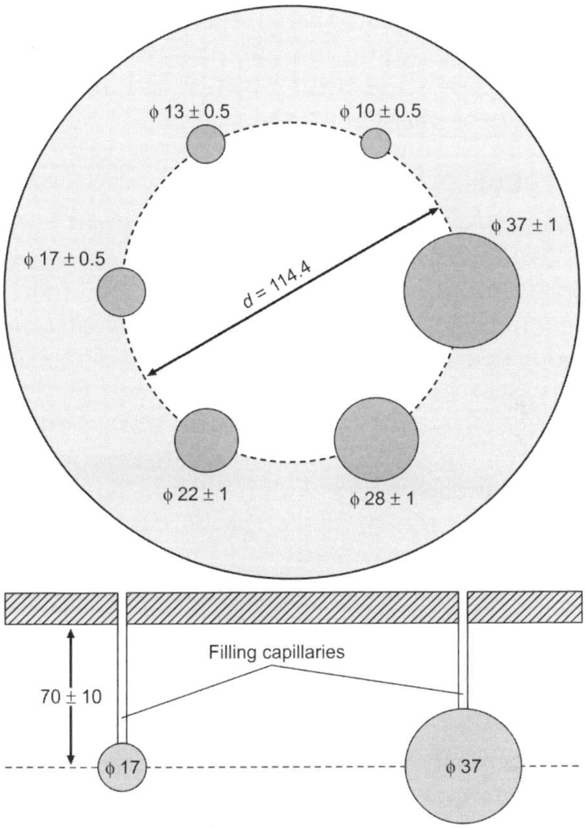

Fig. 2 Phantom insert with hollow spheres

All diameters given are inside diameters. The wall thickness of the spheres shall be less than or equal to 1 mm. The centers of the spheres shall be 70 ±10 mm from the inside surface of the mounting plate so they are axially all in the same transverse slice. Phantom material is polymethylmethacrylate, although the spheres may alternatively be made from glass.

is coplanar to the middle slice of the scanner to within 3 mm throughout the extent of the phantom. A 700 ±5 mm length of the line source of the test phantom shall be filled with 18F and threaded through the 6.4 mm hole in the test phantom. The test phantom shall then be placed at the head end of the body phantom and abutting the body phantom in order to approximate the clinical situation of having activity that extends beyond the scanner.

Data Collection

The data acquisition time shall be determined considering the axial distance, the bed is translated between positions in a total body study (typically less than the axial field-of-view of the scanner) and the total axial imaging distance being simulated. The imaging time shall be set so as to simulate a total body scan, 100 cm total axial imaging distance, in 60 minutes. This time shall include both emission and transmission imaging times assuming attenuation correction is performed at each bed position where distance = 100 cm, and axial step is the distance the bed is moved between positions in a total body study. This time shall include both emission and transmission scan durations, as well as any transition times (e.g. for moving the transmission source or uploading data).

Additional measurements may be taken where the imaging time is increased to simulate a longer total imaging time or a decreased total axial imaging distance. Imaging time that corresponds to a total axial imaging distance of 50 cm in 60 minutes. The actual emission and transmission imaging times are to be reported as well as the total axial imaging distance being simulated. Because the scans have limited counts, it is recommended that 3 replicate scans be acquired in order to improve the reliability of the results. The durations of the subsequent replicate scans should be adjusted for physical decay in order to acquire the same number of events.

Data Processing

All slices shall be reconstructed with all available corrections applied to the data. Images shall be reconstructed using the standard parameters (e.g. image matrix size, pixel size, slice thickness, reconstruction algorithm, filters, or other smoothing applied) for whole-body studies, as recommended by the manufacturer. These reconstruction parameters shall be reported.

Analysis

Image Quality

A transverse image centered on the cold and hot spheres shall be used in the analysis. The same slice shall be used for all spheres. Regions of interest (ROIs) shall be drawn on each hot and cold sphere. A circular ROI shall be used with a diameter as close as possible to the inner diameter of the sphere being measured. The ROI analysis tool should take into account partial pixels and also permit movement of the ROI in increments of 1 mm or smaller.

ROIs of the same sizes as the ROIs drawn on the hot and cold spheres shall be drawn in the background of the phantom on the slice centered on the spheres. Twelve 37 mm diameter ROIs shall be drawn throughout the background at a distance of 15 mm from the edge of the phantom but no closer than 15 mm to any sphere (Fig. 3). ROIs of the smaller sizes (10, 13, 17, 22, and 28 mm) shall be drawn concentric to the 37 mm background ROIs. The ROIs shall also be drawn on the slices as close as possible to ±1 cm and ±2 cm on either side of the central slice. A total of 60 background ROIs of each size, 12 ROIs on each of five slices, shall thus be drawn. The locations of all ROIs shall be fixed between successive measurements (e.g. replicate scans). The average counts in each background ROI shall be recorded.

Frequency of Quality Control Tests

The frequency of QC tests is typically specified along with a test procedure. However, the frequency can be modified by the medical physicist on the basis of the performance and reliability of the equipment, the criticality of the application of the equipment and the results of earlier QC tests.

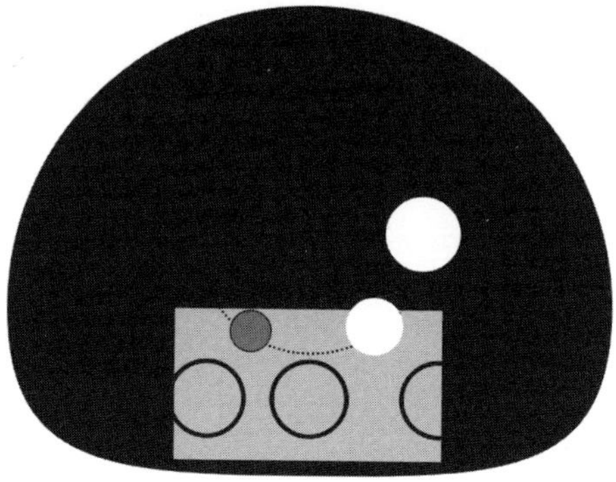

Fig. 3 Background region of interest placement for image quality analysis

Regions of interest (ROIs) shall be drawn on the spheres. The diameters of the ROIs shall be as close as possible to the physical inner diameters of the spheres. In addition, twelve ROIs of each size shall be drawn in the background.

All diagnostic imaging equipment requires a certain amount of calibration, preventive maintenance and component replacement. There is usually no impact on these from QC programmes. When a component fails, it will fail whether it is monitored with a QC programme or not. For example, QCs on the CT photographic processor are almost universally required on a daily basis, before processing any clinical films. However, review of six months of control charts indicates that the monitored values never shift by more than ±0.05 optical density units. Furthermore, all the processing chemicals are mixed in-house in large batches, and each batch of chemicals is tested sensitometrically. Under these conditions, it is acceptable to reduce the frequency of testing, perhaps to one to three times per week, with one test always being carried out before processing of any clinical images at the beginning of the working week. As noted above, the frequency also depends on the criticality of the application. Another example, it is recommended to check the gantry lasers daily. Even though there may not have been any problems with the alignment of the lasers for six months, it is probably not prudent to reduce the frequency of this check if the data are to be used for radiation therapy applications. If there were to be a shift in the laser alignment, this could result in an error in the location of the treatment volume when the images are used for radiation therapy treatment planning. This is a critical application and, therefore, the one for which daily checks are warranted.

The phantom needed for this test is the 'image quality phantom' described in IEC Standard 61675–1, which is also used to assess image quality and accuracy of attenuation and scatter corrections during acceptance testing. The phantom consists of:

(a) A 'body compartment' that is at least 18 cm in interior length in order to cover the whole axial FOV of the PET scanner;
(b) Six hollow spheres with internal diameters of 1.0, 1.3, 1.7, 2.2, 2.8 and 3.7 cm, and a wall thickness of no more than 1 mm;
(c) A cylindrical insert (5.0 ±0.2 cm outer diameter) filled with a material of low atomic number that mimics lung attenuation (average density: 0.3 ±0.1 g/mL), is centred inside the body compartment, and extends axially through the entire phantom. In addition to the image quality phantom, this test requires the use of heavy weights (total weight of about 100 kg) to mimic the

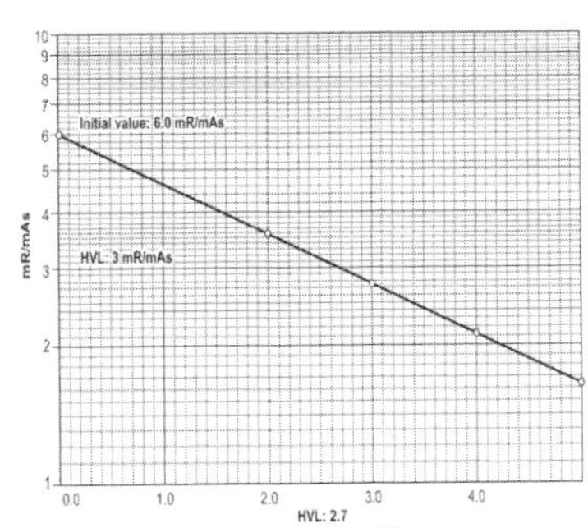

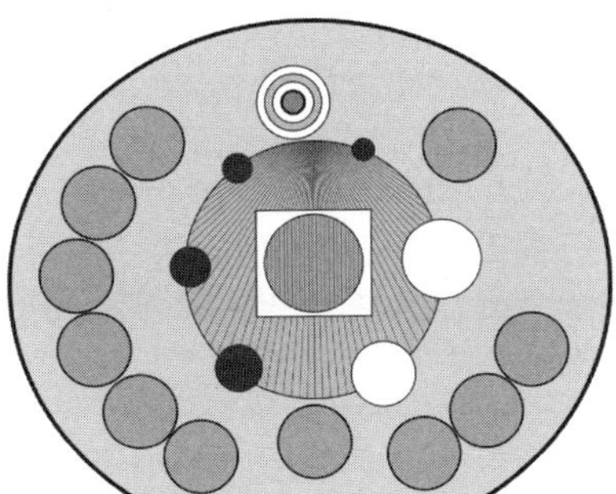

scanning of a heavy patient. Lead bricks or other heavy materials can be used for this purpose.

The body compartment shall be filled with an 18F solution of 5.3 kBq/mL radioactivity concentration. The 2.8 and 3.7 cm spheres shall be filled with cold water to mimic cold lesion imaging. The 1.0, 1.3, 1.7 and 2.2 cm spheres shall be filled with an 18F solution that is 8 times hotter than the background (sphere: background = 8 : 1), i.e. with a concentration of 42.4 kBq/mL. If a lower dose is recommended by the manufacturer for whole body scan, then a lower radioactivity concentration than 5.3 kBq/mL could be used and reported for this test. A practical approach to accurately achieve the 8:1 sphere-to-background ratio without spills is to fill the body compartment with an eighth of its total volume, add the radioactivity intended for the background compartment, use this solution to fill the spheres and then fill the body compartment with water and cover the phantom with the lid to which the spheres are attached. The spheres shall be positioned in such a manner that the centres of all spheres shall be in the same transverse slice, at a 5.72 cm radius from the centre of the phantom, with the 1.7 cm sphere positioned along the horizontal axis of the phantom.The lead bricks (or equivalent heavy weights) shall be uniformly distributed over 1.5 m length of the table adjacent to the quality phantom. The phantom shall be positioned at the end of the table in a supine position. The phantom shall be positioned axially in the scanner so that the centre of the spheres is at the middle slice of the scanner, and positioned transaxially so that the centre of the phantom is centred in the scanner.

The phantom should also be aligned so that the plane through the centres of the spheres is coplanar to the middle slice of the scanner to within 3 mm throughout the length of the phantom. The lead bricks (or equivalent heavy weights) shall be uniformly distributed over 1.5 m length on the table adjacent to the image quality phantom.

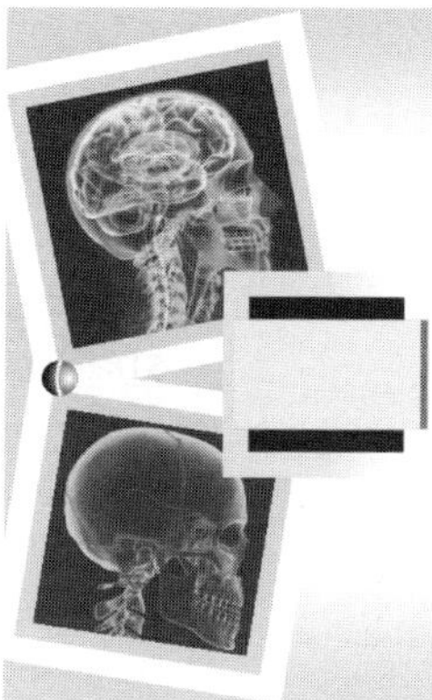

Index